Real M

Paul Stevenson has worke.............................
profitably as a minister, schoolmaster, financial
journalist (in which he still dabbles), sales manager in
Ireland, lecturer in communication, director of a firm
selling metal detectors, investigative radio reporter and
proprietor of a news agency. He is a financial planning
consultant and also does some PR consultancy work.

He lives in Teignmouth with Maureen, his wife of
thirty-four years, and has one daughter, Fiona. Asked
why he had waited so long to publish his first book,
Paul Stevenson said: 'I've been busy.'

Real Medicine

THE A–Z GUIDE

Paul Stevenson

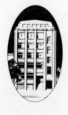

ROBERT HALE · LONDON

ISBN 0 7090 4884 X

Robert Hale Limited
Clerkenwell House
Clerkenwell Green
London EC1R 0HT

Photoset in North Wales by
Derek Doyle & Associates, Mold, Clwyd.
Printed in Great Britain by
St Edmundsbury Press Ltd, Bury St Edmunds, Suffolk.
Bound by WBC Bookbinders Ltd, Bridgend, Glamorgan.

Acknowledgements

My grateful thanks to Trevor Learmouth, of Exeter University Library, for his professional guidance to original sources. Many thanks also to Ian and Elizabeth Cook of Weircliff for their help and encouragement. Finally, I would like to thank the following copyright holders who gave me permission to use quotations from their publications: W.H. Allen, The Ashgrove Press, Elm Tree Books, Hamlyn & Co, Mercier Press and St. Martin's Press.

For Maureen Elizabeth
with all my love forever

Introduction

'Every human being carries in his heart a secret wonderland and nurses the silent longing to find during his lifetime his own North West passage.'

Felix Marti-Ibanez MD, Ed. *The Medical Newsmagazine NY*

A few doors away from one of the country's larger hospitals is a health food shop. All day long the punters file in to out-patients with their lumps, rashes, aches or malfunctions and all day long doctors in white coats listen sympathetically, suggest some tablets or a spot of surgery, and send the punters home feeling better already, despite the fact that while in the waiting room they have probably just contacted enough pathogens to kill a rutting rhinoceros.

But come lunch time, the flow of traffic subtly changes. Doctors, now dressed in civvies, come out of the hospital and into the health food shop where the proprietor, a friend of mine whose main qualification for his prescriptive role is an ability to remember in a nano-second which of his many lines has the highest mark-up, listens professionally to their tales of sorrow with none of the medical hang-ups of a pharmacist who would fear to diagnose or prescribe because he knows that if he did, his professional association would be down on him like a ton of codeine.

David is firm and decisive in both diagnosis and prescription, for he is the true inheritor of the long tradition of Real Medicine, the clamorous voice of uninformed certainty, the lounge bar consultant in super-confident guesswork.

'I've got this sort of tickly cough,' they tell him earnestly, and he listens as attentively as only a health food shop proprietor with high rents to pay can.

'Is it worse in cold weather?' he asks.

'Yes, how did you know that?' they ask, amazed at his powers of

7

perception. 'It sort of tickles when I breathe cold fog. Then I cough.'

He reaches decisively for what I am sure is a random product on his packed shelves: 'Three pound twenty seven for a box of fifteen, right as rain within three or four days, and don't breathe when there's cold fog about,' he says, tapping the keyboard of his computerized till.

'Thank you, thank you,' the doctors gush, and go back on duty with that pleasant inner glow of pharmacoepic security that their prospective patients perched on uncomfortable chairs in endless out-patient queues are still awaiting. The cough clears up within a week or two. They come back and thank him, and buy something else just in case.

To be fair, should my friend the health food shop proprietor feel at all unwell, it would never occur to him to pop any of his own pills. No, David would head straight for the osteopath.

'I've got this sort of tickly cough,' he tells the bone wrencher.

'Is it worse when you breathe cold fog?' he asks, engrossed in the read-out of his new Apple computer spreadsheet and chuckling as the rich pages unfold.

'Yes, how did you know that?' he asks, amazed.

'You've got one leg shorter than the other,' the osteopath tells him, as he tells half his punters: the other half are told that they have one leg longer than the other, a much more expensive problem.

He puts David on his bench, surrounded by very expensive electronic wizardry, and performs two or three traditional wrestling holds on him, in which his head goes one way, his hips the other, and he has his first ever opportunity to look closely at his own buttocks – 'Goodness! Is that what my wife sees each morning when I get out of bed?' – before an agonizing click in his spine triggers spasms of blinding pain. Afterwards, he manages to limp to his wallet and pay cash – please – for the treatment. He gets home, but he is off work for several days. This all shows that the treatment has 'worked'.

Now he just needs to attend three cash sessions a week for a few more months until his inner leg measurements have equalized. The tickly cough, which by now he has forgotten through a miasma of agony and Johnson's Baby Cream, clears up within three or four days. He has spent a lot of money, experienced a lot of pain, and lost a lot of time from work: he has, in other words, received value for money. QE2. (This is similar to QED, but dearer, especially first class in high season, which is how successful osteopaths travel.)

The odd thing is that when David's osteopath feels a tickly cough coming on, worse when he is breathing cold damp air, he goes, not to the health food shop nor to a fellow osteopath, but to the pharmacy round the corner, because he knows the chemist will tell him what he wants to hear, that the reason he has a tickly cough is that he has what doctors call 'a tickly cough' and that the best treatment is a bottle of the same comfortingly sugary cough tincture that his parents used to give him when a child. Should he check with his GP, Justin Case? 'No, no, no,' says the chemist, 'not necessary, not for a tickly cough.'

Pausing only to ask the pharmacist whether he knew that he had one leg longer than the other and giving the now-worried man his business card, the osteopath leaves the dispensary, swigging the familiar lotion with its warm evocation of toasting forks, hot water bottles and the BBC Home Service. The cough clears up within three or four days.

And the chemist? He knows perfectly well that if he does nothing at all his tickly cough will clear up anyway, but he also knows that much of his income is dependent on the good will of the health centre in the next road, so he consults the doctor, who says one of two things to him:

either

'It's too early yet to tell what it is,'

or

'You should have come to me sooner; it's too late now ...'

So where does the primrose-oil path to perfect health lie?

Left to itself, the body is designed to clear up most of life's smaller irritations in about three days, the lesser non-life-threatening conditions inside three weeks, and the more serious ones in about three months. Ask any GP about this rule of three. In the meantime it is well designed to overcome almost any treatment that experts care to inflict on it. Patients are people who feel grateful to whomever it was who did whatever it was that their bodies managed to survive.

This is not to say that modern medicine has not had its stunning successes in treating some very serious conditions. But how would we have managed our day-to-day medical matters had we lived two or three centuries ago, in the days of Real Ale, Real Food and Real Medicine? Read on, kindly bearing in mind the plea of Nich.

Culpeper, Gent, in his original *Herbal*:

> 'They that think the use of these medicines is too brief, it is only for the cheapness of the book.'

A

Acid Belchings

Culpeper's *Complete Herbal* offered an affordable remedy for these uncomfortable and antisocial eructations, though not without awkward consequences at one's place of work:

> Onions are good for cold watery humours, but injurious to people of bilious habit, affecting the head, eyes, and stomach. When plentifully eaten, they procure sleep, help digestion, cure acid belchings, remove obstruction of the viscera, increase the urinary secretions, and promote insensible perspirations.

Aconites

Botanically, the aconite is *Aconitum napellus* or one of its hundred or more relatives throughout the northern hemisphere, a poisonous family of mauve buttercup aka monk's-hood, wolf's-bane and blue rocket. Every part of the plant is dangerous, so much so that for centuries the word 'aconite' was a synonym for 'poison'. The symptoms of aconite poison, according to *Black's Medical Dictionary* of 1951, are similar to those noted in watchers of party political broadcasts: 'The pulse becomes weak, the breathing laboured, and the face livid. Convulsions may come on, but consciousness is retained.'

Some people poisoned themselves by eating aconite in mistake for horseradish, others poisoned themselves in ways that still leave doctors puzzled; just mark something 'poison' and some passer-by will be compelled to drink or eat it. Where was the cure? Nicholas Culpeper's definitive book *The English Physician Enlarged, or the Herbal* of 1653 listed several, including mulberries and a decoction of ground-pine; but with the water supply now profitized, it might be a good idea to stock up on garlic, for this was his favourite way of settling or 'discussing' poisons: 'Garlic has some more peculiar virtues, viz. that it has a special quality to discuss inconveniences, coming by corrupt agues or mineral vapours, or by

11

drinking corrupt and stinking waters; as also by taking wolf-bane, henbane, hemlock, or other poisonous and dangerous herbs.'

The cure was effected by eating the garlic, and two centuries later it is still in the health food shops' top ten herbal panaceas. See also **Treacle, Poor Man's.**

Agues

Strictly, an ague was malaria, but it could mean almost anything. A 'head ague' was probably neuralgia, but shivering colds, leprosy, chicken pox, influenza and scarlatina were all 'agues' of varying severity.

Sir William Paddy (1554-1634) attended King James during an ague that got worse. He was asked to report on the King's health in a letter to the Palace on March 25, 1625[1]: why was he not getting better? Dr Paddy gave four reasons:

1 'The malignity of the ague was the chief malady, and plasters were used several times.
2 King James was an aged person, being sixty years old.
3 He had a plethoric body full of ill humours.
4 the King was adverse to physic and was impatient under it.'

As a counter-irritant, the scalding plasters might well have taken the Royal mind off the Royal ague, but they had no therapeutic value, and the King died twenty-one hours later on 27 March. Paddy wrote:

> Beyng sent for to Thibaulde butt two days before the death of my Soveraigne Lord and master King James: I held it my Christian dutie to prepare hym, telling hym that there was nothing left for me to doe (in ye afternoon of his death ye next day att noone) butt to pray for his soule ... whereunto he cheerfullie accorded.

A kind man and a thoughtful doctor, Paddy comforted his patient and prayed for him. The King, who was understandably impatient with medicine, was cheerful in his acceptance of death.

But what caused agues? What cured them? No-one knew, but ignorance of the facts has never stopped the medical profession from chucking its weight about. One eighteenth-century doctor took a very sniffy view of competing complementary practitioners: 'There is hardly an old woman who is not possessed of a nostrum for stopping an ague; and it is amazing with what readiness their pretensions are believed' said Dr Buchan, Physician to Her Majesty the Queen, with magisterial hauteur in 1784, before listing the orthodox understanding and treatments of the day:

Cause
'Agues are occasioned by effluvia from putrid, stagnating water. [Also] by eating too much stone fruit, a poor watery diet, damp houses, evening dews, watching, fatigue, depressing passions, and the like.'

Prevention of leprosy and smallpox?
'Take care not to be much abroad in wet weather.'

Cures were alcoholic to a degree that puzzles modern clinicians, but wine has probably been in continuous medical use longer than anything else: 'Take of Jamaica pepper, half a pound; of proof spirit, three gallons; of common water, one gallon. Infuse without heat for two or three days, drain off the liquor, then distill off three gallons. This makes an agreeable cordial.'

It is time someone reinvented alcohol therapy, because three gallons of proof spirit at between 57% and 90% alcohol by volume – say twice as strong as whisky – plus one gallon of water, distilled down to a quarter of its volume and drunk as a cordial must have killed almost every known germ or bacillus, and dulled a lot of pain.

Agues & Snake Root Specials
Even better, when patients had a mega-ague they might have tried one of Dr Buchan's appealingly-named Snake Root specials:

> Take a drachm of Peruvian bark [Cinchona bark, from which quinine is made]; Virginian snake-root, and orange peel, of each half an ounce; bruise them all together, and infuse for five or six days in a bottle of brandy, Holland gin, or any good spirit; afterwards, pour off the clear liquor, and take a wine glass twice or thrice a day.

Snake root was the root of American milkwort (*Polygala senega*), believed by the Seneca Indians to be helpful when treating snake bites. However, Nicholas Culpeper of herbal fame believed that only English plants could cure English ills; after all, he reasoned closely, why would the stars give you an illness in Devon and put the cure in North America? It made no astrological sense to him at all.

Dr Buchan's turbo-potcheen may have been the original of that nice little pharmaceutical earner, the repeat prescription, despite his discordant caveat that feverish agues could be caused by 'fleeping in the fun, eating spiceries, and drinking ftrong liquor'.

This need to state the obvious about sunburn continues: *The Side Effects Book* by Dr Trevor Smith, published in 1989 contains this strangely similar advice: 'Where a barrier-cream protection is not used, extensive deep burns can occur, sometimes after falling asleep in the sun.'

To balance his alcoholic prescriptions, Dr Buchan also recommended, in comfortingly inscrutable medical language:

> A regimen to dilute the blood, correct the acrimony of the humours, allay the excessive heat, remove the spasmodic strictures of the vessels, and promote the secretions ... infusions of bitter herbs, as camomile, wormwood, or water trefoil; gentian root or centaury ... sometimes a scruple to a dram of powdered ipecacuanha is sufficient for an adult as a vomit, then give weak camomile tea to drink.

The standard back-up treatment for agues, fevers or almost anything at all was to open a vein with a razor and draw off half a bucket of blood. This was not as simple as it might sound, because before they could open a vein the surgeon first had to ask some searching questions: date of birth, star sign, today's date, and position of all major planets (except Pluto, which had not yet been spotted by scientists and could not therefore rejig anybody's DNA). Only then could he be sure that a blood exfusion was astrologically indicated:

> Bleeding is of the greatest importance. This operation should be performed as soon as the symptoms of a fever appear.
> A person suffers from an Ague when he has bad blood. He should be cut as soon as the moon passes through the middle of Gemini and bled until good blood appears. If the blood is black, draw it off until red blood appears. If the blood ceases to flow, the wound can be opened again with the tip of a finger.

One hopes that he was not looking for arterial blood in a vein, or the patient could be in for a really bad time. Robin Hood is widely believed to have been bled to death by a witch who deliberately left him to empty at a session such as this. The standard fee was one shilling a go.

Agues – The Herbal Route

The lodestone of the herbalists, Nicholas Culpeper[2], set out in the seventeenth century to codify and anglicise the experience of more than two thousand years' development in herbal treatments. He still has his followers today, though they are selective rather than faithful followers – see Culpepper on **Colic** for one of his less popular nostrums. For agues he suggested that:

> An ounce of gentian root, calamus aromaticus, and orange peel, of each half an ounce, with three or four handfuls of camomile flowers, and an handful of coriander seed, all bruised together in a mortar, may be used in the form of an infusion or tea. About half an handful of these ingredients may be put into a teapot, and an English pint of boiling water poured on them. Three or four cups a day is the dose.

And why not? It must have been safer than being cut with a greasy razor, but his rationality twitched a little when he slipped into astrological mode in this professional plug for cinquefoil (*Potentilla*):

> Let Jupiter be angular and strong when gathered: and if you give but a scruple (which is but twenty grains) of it at a time, either in white wine or white wine vinegar, you shall seldom miss the cure of an ague, be it what ague soever, in three fits, as I have often proved to the admiration of myself and others.

To be fair, though, the old self-publicist used the word 'admiration' in its earlier sense of 'wonder at' rather than in its modern clinical sense of 'calling a press conference.'

He also ridiculed one then current cure for a feverish ague – 'drinking large quantities of strong liquors and jumping in rivers'. There are modern practitioners who would endorse this scepticism.

Almonds in the Ears
It is always dangerous to be complacent, so the fact that this painful illness is no longer with us is no reason to remain ignorant of the fact that it could be cured, according to Culpeper's *Herbal* by Devil's Bit or Hedge Mustard.

Alternative Therapies
Lest we think that there is today a medical orthodoxy that replaces all ancient recipes and prescriptions, it is worth noting that when Brian Inglis and Ruth West in 1983 brought out a guide to alternative therapies[3] – votes of no confidence – they had no difficulty in filling their pages: Rolfing, Naturopathy, Hydrotherapy, Ionization therapy, Bakes Eyesight Training, Tissue salts therapy, Herbalism, Aroma therapy, Bach Flower Remedies, Homeopathy, Anthroposophy, Osteopathy, Cranial Osteopathy, Chiropractic, the Alexander Principle, Feldenkrais Technique, Reflexology, Applied Kinesiology, Acupuncture, Shiatsu, Yoga, T'ai Chi, Aikido, Dance therapy, Colour therapy, Music therapy, Hypnotherapy, Couéism, Silva Mind Control, Autogenic Training, Meditation, Biofeedback, Dream therapy, Behaviour therapy, Rogerion therapy, Encounter therapy, Gestalt, Psychodrama, Transactional Analysis, Co-Counselling, Bioenergetics, Reichian therapy, Polarity therapy, Metamorphic Technique, Rebirthing and Psychosynthesis.

It is quite feasible that since 1983 even more alternative and complementary approaches to health and fitness have developed. See also **Ramsden Therapy**, or **Ramsdenism**.

Amatory Problems, Mainly in Men
Mankind, and to a much lesser extent womankind, has always been in the market for aphrodisiacs. Thousands of them have been marketed over thousands of years and yet man's restless quest for more nooky continues. Why keep searching when earlier centuries abounded with orthodox and paramedical potions, like this one of Culpeper's? 'Dragon's blood never fails.'

Where could they get a supply of dragons' blood after Lancelot had recklessly depredated this endangered species? Dragon's blood was a red resin taken from a big tree found on the Canaries – *Dracaena draco*, of the Lileaceae. In these unromantic days we use it for making varnishes; Culpeper dissolved it and drank it, importing a lasting gloss to the male libido.

The key to formulating aphrodisiacs was to understand how the reproductive process worked. Hippocrates had shown by a simple experiment of his that cutting off a man's testicles – another man's, not his own – reduced his ability to perform. What did this prove? 'On sperm and its production opinions vary. Galen said that blood descends from all the organs and is changed from red into white sperm: Hippocrates said that the change is made in the brain and that the sperm descends to the testicles, for when they are cut no one can produce it.'

Following this interesting line of scientific reasoning, a psychosexual counsellor researching for his doctorate at the university of Ongar spent some decades training a team of spiders to respond to spoken commands.

Eventually he reached the stage where he could place them in a line on the far side of the slide, and know that when he said 'Come!' they would scamper obediently towards him across the glass and that on the command 'Go!' they would turn round and scamper back to the other side.

However, after demonstrating this acquired ability a sufficient number of times to convince his peers that more than coincidence was involved, he took the experiment a stage further by pulling off all their legs, and now when he said, 'Come!' the spiders did not move! This, he argued to his engrossed colleagues, proved that spiders hear the human voice through their feet. There was general agreement and he was soon awarded his doctorate in Arachnid Audiometry. He still successfully practices in downtown Ongar.

Amatory Problems & Pepper
Why do pubs whose only food is microwaved lasagna, chilli con carne or curry still put pepper pots on the tables? Could it be because publicans retain deep and ancient folk memories of its hidden qualities that might help their customers in their nooky-quest? 'The

seed [of *Sinapsis Nigra*], taken either in an electuary or drink, stirs up lust, and helps the gnawings of the bowels. The decoction of the black pepper seed made in wine and drank, resists poisons, the malignity of mushrooms, and the bites of venomous creatures, if taken in time.'

Amatory Problems – Gaining Power over Women

There were both moral and medical reasons for not indulging in sexual orgies at times of ill-health. In his article 'The manuscript lecture notes of Alexander Monro primus', historian D W Taylor included this observation from Monro's 1725 lecture notes: 'All acts of venery are to be shunned for these increase the circulation much at the time and ennervate afterwards ... a young man who was wounded in the head with a fractyure in the scull, after 5 weeks when the wound was almost cicatrised, by lying with his miss fell into a fever and died.' One has to admire a lad who could undertake such an exercise with a fractured skull, but the medical point is taken.

According to McGrew's *Encyclopedia of Medical History*, carrots were long believed to be powerful aphrodisiacs – look at rabbits – and much more interestingly, that 'Fern seed spores gave men power over women.' You have been warned. Carrots held a similar power, possibly by helping jaded men to realize that not all cats are grey in the dark.

Apoplexy

Apoplexy [Greek: a sudden stroke] was invented by Hippocrates and it meant a diseased condition of the brain that caused sudden insensibility or bodily disablement, so it follows that an apoplectic person could not be angry.

What did Real Medicine doctors do when patients presented with apoplexy? The author of the thirteenth-century text book, *Practica*, knew his limitations and set them out in print, to the chagrin of his bank manager: 'Let the reader note that I do not deal with certain affections, such as epilepsy, chronic toothache, paralysis, apoplexy, etc., because I think they are incurable.' While there was no cure, relief did eventually arrive in the form of nature's general anaesthetic, death.

The herbal recipe was to take flowers of lily of the valley, extract the juice, set it to ferment in a sealed jar in dung for a few months, and then apply the resultant liquor externally. This cured apoplexy. Walnuts had a similar effect.

Apothecaries

There has always been a strict pecking order in the medical world, starting with physicians (first division), then surgeons (second division), and finally apothecaries (Gr. *apotheke*, a warehouse), who were firmly set in the third division as a sort of inferior doctor who had not quite made it. Herbalists, mainly elderly women, were well down in the amateur ranks.

In England during the eighteenth and early nineteenth centuries apothecaries and surgeons had to renounce membership of their own qualifying bodies before they could become licentiates of the Royal College of Physicians. In Scotland's more enlightened milieu, medics were studying pharmacy along with chemistry, botany and midwifery as early as 1739, neatly combining the main disciplines in one qualification, while picking up four sets of fees.

Women had always been accepted as members of the lowly Society of Apothecaries, provided only that they completed an apprenticeship in their ancient art; this reflected foreign established practice that had been imported into England along with the Norman conquest, whereby women practiced medicine 'from castle to cottage,' preparing herbal remedies, fixing fractures, dressing wounds and generally first-aiding. Indeed, this involvement of women in domestic medicine and their making up of simple but effective local prescriptions may well have led to the black propaganda campaign that called their practical work 'old wives' tales'.

Apothecaries' Weights

The British have never been happy with standardized weights and measures, seeing them as some kind of challenge to the ingrained national eclecticism that is reflected in our landscape, our architecture and our langauge. We started by importing the Roman sixteen-ounces-to-the-pound system, but called it 'avoirdupois' to confuse the French, who are still trying to find an equivalent term in their language. Then Henry III passed an Act in 1266 that pleased his subjects' love of the absurd by decreeing that: 'An English penny called the sterling, round and without clipping, shall weigh thirty-two grains of wheat, well dried and gathered out of the middle of the ear, and twenty pence (pennyweights) do make an ounce and twelve ounces a pound, and eight pounds do make a gallon of wine, which is the eighth of a quarter.'

This left apothecaries sucking their quills thoughtfully as they tried to make sense of doctors' prescriptions, and heaven only knows what Brussels would have said. Edward I hardly helped in 1304 with his statute that tried to simplify matters in the English tradition of being innovative without changing anything, radical without upsetting anybody, and decisive while keeping one's options open: 'Every pound of money or of medicines is of twenty shillings weight, but the pound of all things is twenty-five shillings weight; the ounce of medicines consists of twenty pence, and the pound contains twelve ounces, but in other things the pound contains fifteen ounces, in both cases the ounce weighing twenty pence.'

With the pound now weighing exactly twelve, fifteen or sixteen ounces, the apothecary looked wearily abroad for some rationality and found it, as we all did in 1969, in France. There, in the town of Troyes, was held a distinguished international fair where coins – frequently pared to the point of mutilation – were sold by weight rather than by face value. Although French, this looked like a good idea.

Sir Theodore Turquet de la Mayerne adopted the Troy standard for the Royal College of Physicians' Pharmacopoeia in 1618, but the sixteen-ounce pound continued alongside it, inadvertently giving rise to the look of dumb misapprehension with which customers to this day hand over their prescriptions to be made up. It was even worse in the United States of America, where the British standards for both troy and avoirdupois were adopted in 1836, but with their own home-grown gallon retained in the interests of confusion.

No wonder apothecaries and others rejoiced when the Mother of Parliaments legalized the metric system in 1864: it could only be months, they reasoned, before the metric system replaced this anarchic assembly of grains and ounces and pounds, and neither was it, in a sense, for a century is not so long a time in politics.

The traditional apothecary's measures were:

20 grains	= 1 scruple
3 scruples	= 1 drachm
8 drachms	= 1 pound

60 minims	= 1 fluid drachm
8 fluid drachms	= 1 fluid ounce (28.412 millilitres)
16 fluid ounces	= 1 pint
8 pints	= 1 gallon

Apothecaries, like pharmacists, were very careful over their measurements, whereas herbal and domestic practitioners depended on broader terms like a 'cup' (about eight fluid ounces), a tablespoon (about half a fluid ounce), and a 'drop' (about one minim): the 'about' was the cause for concern when the medicine being dispensed was raw opium or the long-popular quicksilver, in which case a drop approximated to the length of a piece of string in terms of the harm that could be inflicted.

To this day, gold, silver and other precious metals are traded on the Exchange in troy ounces.

Appetite

France, which gave us the aperitif, once railed against taking wine with meals. The *Mémoires de la Société Royale de Médecine*[4], made this astonishing claim in 1806: 'By drinking at proper times, thirst will be prevented at improper times, and we shall have no temptation to fill the stomach with liquids when we take our food, thus setting it afloat, and diluting the juices of the stomach, upon the agency of which its digestion entirely depends.'

Dr Buchan was unimpressed; he still recommended Bitter Wine aperitif: 'Take of gentian root, yellow rind of lemon peel, fresh, each one ounce; long pepper, two drams; mountain wine, two pints. Infuse without heat for a week and strain out the wine for use. Take a glass before dinner and supper.'

Appetite – Stopping Women's for Unusual Meats
The medlar, *mespilus Germanicus*, was recommended by Culpeper for all fathers-to-be who wished to cut down on their Sainsbury's bill during those critical craving months. Significantly, our local Sainsbury's does not stock medlars. 'The fruit, if eaten by pregnant women, stops their longings for unusual meats.' Medlars you can grow: fromage frais with grilled kiwi's legs you cannot.

Appetite – Curing Loathing of Meat
Vegetarian daughters who yukked at the dinner table could be cured, if only their parents could persuade them to take the remedy seriously: 'If a poultice or plaster be made with dried medlars, beaten and mixed with the juice of red roses, whereunto a few cloves and nutmegs may be added, and a little red coral also, and applied to the stomach that is given to loathing meat, it will effectually help.' Worth a try, surely?

Appetite – Indulging Women's Depraved
Dr Buchan suggested that spoiling pregnant women, even depraved ones, might be medically acceptable, but only within strict limits: 'Every woman with child ought to be kept cheerful and easy in her mind. Her appetite, though depraved, ought to be indulged as far as prudence will permit.' Prudence was probably her mother-in-law.

Arteries
Arteries were for long believed to contain air (artery – a windpipe) mixed with vital spirits and some blood. The heart sucked air in through the lungs and the pores of the skin, then pushed out 'fulliganous vapours', a sort of smoke from the burning food in the guts. The liver, of course, produced the blood that ebbed and flowed through the body.

Then William Harvey discovered in 1628 what really happened. Blood, he discovered, circulated through the arteries in one direction only, then soaked into the tissue through pores in the flesh and oozed

back through other pores into the veins. And so on. Many
haematologists are no longer convinced that he was right about this,
but generously give him the credit for discovering the principle of
circulation.

Culpeper saw veins and arteries as a cosmetic problem when they
went wrong. He had two remedies: one was to rub the juice of a Blue
Bottle onto the affected area, Blue Bottle being, of course, the blue
cornflower, a weed of the Compositae (*Centaurea Cyanus*); the other
was to apply Clown's woundwort, otherwise marsh woundwort, of
the genus Stachys.

Asthma

Asthma had as many putative remedies as did agues. Like today's
treatments, most were harmless, and some were even helpful in
treating the distressing symptoms. Real Medicine used whatever was
in the garden: Boil some fresh nettles in a pan over the fire, and let
them simmer. Strain off the liquor, and drink when cool. Set fire to
some well-dried nettles and breath in the smoke. Boil some onions,
and as they cool, mix honey into the warm onion juice and give some
to the sufferer to drink.

Some radical souls linked asthma to lifestyle. When Archbishop
Hamilton called the Italian specialist Geronimo Cordano to
Edinburgh in 1552 to cure his asthma, he was disappointed to be told
to overcome his breathing difficulty by exercising, going out in the
fresh air and also by ceasing forthwith his custom of '... having a
woman every night before and after supper.'

According to Roderick McGrew's *Encyclopedia of Medical
History*, Scottish doctors were furious with this totally irrelevant
attack on ecclesiastical privilege – what could such practices possibly
have to do with breathlessness in an overweight middle-aged
archbishop? – and accused Cordano of witchcraft, the medieval
equivalent of being struck off. The archbishop, however, paid up and
offered Cordano a retainer to stay on in Edinburgh and come up with
some more novel ideas. Cordano declined, perhaps preferring to wait
until Calvin had put forward broadly similar views of his own on
theological grounds some seven years later. The women of
Edinburgh sighed with relief and got back to their knitting.

Convulsive and Periodic asthmas were discussed at length by Dr
Thomas Willis in 1670. The sufferer, he decided, must get used to
foreign lager – and keep a bucket handy:

> In those diseases I have found nothing more efficacious than that the
> patient should once or twice a month consume large quantities of milky
> beer with uncooked leaves of Thistle, and that then vomiting should be
> induced by a feather or finger thrust into the throat; this must be
> repeated many times.

The serum of the blood is to be drawn off at suitable times by Diaphoretics or Diuretics. For this reason the use of millipedes is often wont to be effective; and frequently help is afforded by tincture of tartar salt, salt of amber, and flowers of Armonic salt.[5]

The millipedes were eaten whole – they had a 'saltish' flavour – or they could be dried and powdered to be available as diuretics when out of season. Not in current use.

The old wives' common treatment for asthma was to roll up some dried coltsfoot into a cigarette and smoke it. (No letters from Pony Club members, please; coltsfoot in this context is *tussilago Farfara*, a composite plant with large soft leaves rather than large soft eyes.) Much relief resulted.

Culpeper recommended herbal decoctions of angelica, bay tree, beans (French), calamine, hound's tongue, lavender, rosemary, garden thyme and masterwort, yet asthma lingers tormentingly on.

If the coughing refused to yield to any of these methods, vomiting could be induced with briony root (*Bryonia dioica*) from the hedgerow, crushed to a powder and mixed with a drop of asaret (foul-smelling Persian gum resin). This latter prescription dates from the twelfth century[6], so at least it had been adequately tested.

Atribiliary Mania

Atribiliary mania, or black bile disease, was one of those vague disorders that doctors could profitably write learned papers about, and in Paris in 1806[7], M Michel Hallé did just that: he explained what was 'wrong' with the patient, and what treatment would 'work' in effecting a 'cure': 'The patient has dropsy, hypochondriasis, accompanied by difficulty of breathing and palpitation, an obstinate cough and, [I paraphrase] an overall glumness.'

Since this typical case of atribiliary mania had been brought on by a surfeit of black bile in the stomach and bowels, the treatment, Dr Hallé reasoned, was to 'Empty the stomach and bowels of black bile with a firm purge '*par la mélange des purgatifs résineux et des mercuriaux,*' for this mania is a disorder of function, and not a disease of structure.' It sounded much more convincing in French.

B

Barbers

Barbers were granted a royal charter from King Edward IV to practise surgery as the 'Mystery of Barbers of London' in 1462, a privilege that orthodox 'short coat' surgeons had to envy for a further thirteen years. Only in 1745 did an Act of Parliament separate surgeons from barbers. The last recorded barber-surgeon was a Mr Middleditch, of Great Suffolk Street, Borough, who practised hairdressing, surgery, bleeding and dentistry until his death in 1821, since when little or nothing has been heard from him.

From Roman times barbers had run health clubs offering bleeding, hair styling, herniotomies (which implied castration at no extra charge), cataract removal, enemas-for-pleasure, tooth-pulling, cupping, kidney-stones-removed-while-you-wait, shaving and the usual surgeons' snipping off of unconsidered trifles.

Chaucer recorded the fact that barber-surgeons not only 'let blood and clipped and shaved' but also drew up legal contracts and conveyances, thereby fulfilling every Jewish mother's dream – 'My son the doctor *and* lawyer.' In 1542 Parliament granted them exemption from bearing arms or serving on juries, so important were their professional services deemed to be.

But how good were these early Sassoons at operating on diseased limbs and organs when not primping? As late as 1743 there were still 300 registered barber-surgeons in Paris alone and if all, or even most, of their customers had died of septicaemia or haemorrhage, would they have successfully traded over such a long period? Yet who today goes to a barber for, say, a light trim and herniotomy?

It is generally said that the barber's pole owes it origin to the barber-surgeons, but this is only half-true. Both barber-surgeons and the High Street bleeding shops traditionally gave their customers a pole to grasp in order to stimulate the flow of blood, and the barber-surgeons kept a supply of bandages rolled around the pole. When not in use the pole was hung at the door as a sign. However, there was perceived to be a need to distinguish the barber-surgeons from the common bleeding shops, as Lord Thurlow pointed out when addressing the House of Lords in July, 1797:

> By a statute, still in force, barbers and surgeons were each to use a pole [as a shop sign]. The barbers were to have theirs blue and white, striped, with no other appendage; but the surgeons', which was to be the same in other respects, was likewise to have a gully-pot and a red rag, to denote the particular nature of their vocations.

So barbers have no right at all to their red and white striped poles. As hospitals compete more and more for their business, surgeons might see some merit in clamouring for their exclusive right to hoist the red and white pole outside their operating theatres, and thereby attracting in some passing trade. The law is on their side.

Barrenness
Buchan expressed the mainstream orthodox, scientific, naggingly professional view: 'Barrenness results frequently from high living, which vitiates the humours. We should imitate the life of the peasants with their simple regimen and their long hours of wholesome exercise. The peasant does not suffer from barrenness or impotence, therefore if we imitate his life we shall have large families, too.'

Surely this is not why the middle classes go in for gardening, jogging, cycling and other peasant occupations? And was country life truly all thatched bliss and roses? Dr Buchan had said on the record in 1778: 'Almost one half of the human species perish in infancy, by improper care and neglect.'

Dr Taylor of Croydon was known in the 1780s as 'The Milk Doctor'[8] because 'he brought several families to childbirth' by a strict diet of milk and vegetables. His fame spread, and even that famed walker, Dr Cheyne, took up the simple cause: 'Eschew all foods but vegetables, all drink save milk.'

Did it 'work'? Of course it did, until some calculating sceptics – possibly journalists – started recording the results objectively instead of anecdotally, when the magic turned sour like unused milk. Interest drooped, like a languid parsnip, as disillusioned people gave it up and waited for something else to come along and re-illusion them. There was always something else.

Bath Waters
Were the Bath waters therapeutic or psychosomatic? Orthodox or quackery? Was Mr Joseph Hume Spry[9] a physician or a bought and paid for hack when, earning his living promoting Bath waters (always expressed in the plural to avoid the risk of people going home and

ladling scented suds down their throats), he wrote a learned work two hundred years ago claiming that they had a role in curing uterine disorders, paralysis and lead colic?

If he was no more than a quack, what are we to say of his contemporary, Dr Edward Barlow MD, physician of Bath Hospital, and his similar work[10], plugging Bath waters for the treatment of gout, rheumatism, palsy and eruptive diseases? Or today's NHS patients still being sent for a Bath bath by their doctors?

The only justification for a trip to this traffic-ridden resort of hot, smelly waters and cold, sullen beggars more recently was the Pump Room string quartet, whose talented players took it in turns to leave the stage for the lavatory every fifteen minutes and was therefore functionally a trio, but a delightful trio. See also **Piffing by Drops**.

Bed-Wetting

The wise Dr Wesley, of Methodism fame, helped parents in many ways in those innocent days before social workers learned to abseil down from assault helicopters to arrest unsuspecting infants at dawn and put them in institutions where they could be buggered by qualified staff. Wesley knew why a child wet the bed: 'he only does it to annoy, because he knows it teases.' As an experienced rural traveller, he was no doubt familiar with the obnoxious clamminess of pre-wetted beds, and had a cure that was as sound and firm as a Devon apple: To Cure Bed-Wetting in a Child. Give the child nothing to drink.

Incidentally, City folk say that investing in gilts is rather like wetting the bed: at first it gives you a warm, comfortable feeling, but you know that sooner or later you will have to get out.

Belly, Ileus

Dr Robert Thornton[11] gave his patients clear instructions for pains of the belly, whether caused by ileus [knotted bowels], incarcerated hernia, or obstinate costiveness [constipation]. The only possible side-effect was some difficulty in giving it up when the illness had subsided:

> The smoke of burning tobacco [is] to be thrown into the anus with great advantage. The smoke operates here by the same qualities that are in the infusion mentioned above; but as the smoke reaches further into the intestines than injections can commonly do, it is thereby applied to a larger surface, and may therefore be a more powerful medicine than the infusions. In several instances, however, I have been disappointed of its effects, and have been obliged to have resort to other means.

Bellows can still be obtained from second-hand shops and junk stalls; ask whether they are VAT-free if intended for medical use – but think carefully before resorting to this treatment without professional advice.

Belly – Opening and Closing the

Culpeper had much to say about the belly, a portmanteau term, as it were, for almost everything below the diaphragm and above the knees. Mainly he listed binders and openers of the belly: 'Binders of the Belly: Holly, Knapweed, Mulberry-tree, Peach-tree, Rose (damask). Openers of the belly: All-Heal, Cabbages, Holly, Lady's Smock, Marsh Mallows (common), Peach tree, Plums, Rhubarb (great monk's).'

A decoction of the tops of hops (*Humulus Lupulus*) did everyone a power of good: 'Open obstructions of the liver and spleen, cleanse the blood, loosen the belly, clear the reins of gravel, and provoke urine.'

But the 'most powerful opener' was wild garlic roots: 'it seldome agrees with dry constitutions, but it performs almost miracles in phlegmatic habits of body.'

Belly – Fluxes of the

So successful were some of the ancient Real Medicines that the illnesses they treated no longer exist – like Culpeper's[19] herbal cure for Fluxes of the Belly: 'Honey Wort (*Cerinthe Major*) or the Greater Honey Wort grows upon a thick green stock to a moderate height. It springs in April, flowers May to August, and perishes in winter. The juice of the herb, with a little saffron dissolved in it, is an excellent remedy.'

It was equally good for 'promoting women's courses', and, by a curious pharmaceutical conjunction, for 'weak, watery, bleared eyes.'

Bilious Attacks

Culpepper was clear in 1660: for the bilious, a simple drink of redcurrants with [diuretic] dandelions and [laxative] sorrel leaves, infused together, did the trick. Why has today's revived interest in Real Medicine not led people back to the hedgerows and cottage gardens for the real thing? Why has it rather led people into expensive shops that charge high prices for the dried up or powdered traces of plants that probably died and went to the factory for processing and packing ages ago. Why?

For example, if parents could not tell whether a child was really too sick to go to school, or just too sick of school to go, Dr Buchan's *Domestic Medicine Modernized* of 1808 offered a solution that could have been made up in any garden shed: 'Take a red currant drink for bilious attacks, or dandelion [diuretic, hence 'Piss-a-Bed'] with sorrel leaves. Millipedes [laxative] can be eaten, though they are said to taste saltish; either whole, as a powder, or their expressed juice.'

Bites, esp. of Shrew-Mice
Stephen Brasnell, in 1633, suggested some therapeutic revenge on creatures that bit or stung:

> The flesh of the same beast that biteth, inwardly taken, helpeth much, and outwardly the best thing to be applied is the flesh of the same beast that did the hurt, pounded in a morter and applied in manner of a poultis.
>
> Now the shrew-mouse is a little kind of mouse with a long sharpe snout and a short tayle; it liveth commonly in old ruinous walls. It biteth also very venomously, and leaveth foure small perforations made by the foure foreteeth. To cure her biting, her flesh roasted and eaten is the best inward antidote if it may be had. And outwardly apply her warme liver and skin if it may be had. Otherwise, Rocket-reeds beaten into a powder, and mixed with the bloud of a dog. Or els the teeth of a dead man made into a fine powder.

All of which could have been bought at the local Tesco's.

Blindness
Worms and teething were held to be a primary cause of blindness (or extreme short-sightedness) in children, as Dr Brisbane's observations[20] show:

> 'I allude to the effects of the irritability of teething upon the health of children. The brain is sometimes so affected as to cause convulsions; the digestive organs are almost constantly disordered. The appetite fails, the tongue is furred; the secretions of the liver are either suspended, diminished or vitiated. There is also a troublesome cough. Such symptoms generally subside when the local irritation ceases ... The motion of a worm in the stomach produces temporary blindness or convulsions.'

Had you known a phlebotomist who was also an astrological consultant, you could confidently have waved your spectacles goodbye: 'If you let blood on April 11 or March 17 you will not suffer blindness.'[21]

Blindness – Wesley's Shocking Discovery
Dr Wesley, always on the lookout for health tips, was thrilled to find a new scientific gadget that could eliminate blindness, tapeworms and

epilepsy with one short, sharp shock. In 1760[22] he announced, as 'a Lover of mankind', that electricity could now cure 'blindness, depression, epilepsy, paralysis, convulsions, hysterical attacks, tapeworms, blindness and tooth aches.[22]

Psychiatrists have since discovered that they can cause some interesting convulsions with few if any traceable deaths by blasting their patients' brains with electric discharges, but Dr Wesley had already been there. He stumbled upon the 'Triboelectric Generator', a glass cylinder machine made by Edward Nairne in 1782 and sold as the 'Insulated Medical Electrical Machine.'

What did this 'miracle machine' do? Briefly, it did for patients' bodies what ECT does for their brains. The amount of high potential charge generated depended on the size of the prime conductor, or on the Leyden jar accumulating the generated charge, so doctors could experiment across the whole range from a light toasting to a total microwave. One exciting byte of data was that the users allegedly experienced an increase in their pulse rate from 80 up to 85 or 90 per minute, and this was clearly a good thing; later research attributed this boost to the victims' near-hysterical tension as they awaited their turn in Dr Wesley's electric chair.

Did it 'work', though? The patient was placed in an insulated chair and connected to the prime conductor of the electrical machine by means of a stout copper wire or chain. He – for it was usually a he – was then electrified positively, although he could sometimes be charged negatively for a change. Being thus 'surrounded by an electrical atmosphere' he was having an 'electric bath' – which was clearly good for him because it was new, and it stimulated the flow of vital spirits from his soul to his body through his recently discovered nerve tubes. That had to be good for him.

The treatment was repeated daily for an hour. During the electrification process, sparks could be drawn off from the patient by means of earthed copper spheres to prove that it 'worked' and that he was getting value for money. Any increase in the size of the spheres would mean an increase in the shock – and in the bill.

Like blood exfusions, the whole thing seemed unlikely, yet it 'worked' as well as ECT ever did, and it caught on because few if any patients died within a sueable distance of the surgery. It had a bitter critic in the Dutch scientist Van Marum, but once again marketing skills outweighed clinical research.

Blindness – When Caused by Great Toads
An account written in the 1630s showed that sometimes animals could strike back at exploiting humans:

Myself, while a student at Cambridge, was so hurt by the spouting of a venomous humour from the body of a great toad into my face while I pashed him to death with a brickbat. Some of the moisture lighted on my right eye, which did not a little endanger it, and hath made it ever since apt to receive any flux of Rheume or Inflammation.

And serve him right for pashing the toad in the first place.

Blisters

Causing a blister as a counter-irritant to inflammation elsewhere is an ancient form of amusement among doctors: it meant that instead of having a stomach ague, they could have a stomach ague *and a blister*. The 1948 edition of *Black's Medical Dictionary*[24] described the process:

> These are employed in cases of both acute and chronic inflammation, on the principle that irritation of the skin causes congestion of the parts immediately below the skin, while it relieves congestion of deep-seated organs through an action upon the nerves that regulate the size of the minute blood vessels.
>
> The chief rubefacients [substances that redden the skin and cause it to peel off] are: mustard, turpentine, cajuput oil, capsicum, tincture of iodine, and liniments of ammonia, chloroform, etc, and of vesicants [substances that cause blisters; a rubefacient becomes a vesicant if it is left on for too long] we have cantharides or Spanish fly, pure acetic acid, ammonia, and chloroform.

Medical science would have agreed with Black two hundred years ago, but Dr Buchan also knew that cantharides, or Spanish fly, was a good external treatment for 'paralytic affections, dropsies, stoppage of urine, asthmatic cases, some of which were very longstanding, and in hysterical disorders.'

Dr Thornton, however, kept his finger on the pulse of medical fashion when he reflected that since opium was easily grown in the garden, was freely available at low prices, and gave the punters an immediate effect that they could talk about down the pub, it should be more widely used. This was his modish prescription[25] for dealing with painful blisters: 'Take two poppy heads, boil them in a quart of milk, and use this as a fomentation. Excellent in inflamed eyes, used also to relieve the pain of inflammation from a blister or other cause.'

Blood

There has always been something special about blood. The Bible mentions it over 400 times. It forbade the eating of blood, or the eating of animals that had not been bled, but the prohibition was moral and symbolic rather than dietary: 'You shall not partake of the blood of any flesh, for the life of all flesh is its blood. Anyone who partakes of it shall be cut off.' (Leviticus 13:14, Tanakh translation.)

This was contrary to the general view of the time, because for 2,000 years 'blood was regarded as the sovereign remedy for leprosy' in ancient Egypt. King Esar-haddon of Assyria, a country then famed for its medical expertise, called in the doctors when his son contracted the disease: 'The prince is doing much better; the king, my lord, can be happy. Starting with the 22nd day I give him blood to drink, he will drink it for three days. For three more days I shall give him blood by internal application.'

The first council of the early Christians reduced Moses' Law to four edicts, two of which had to do with blood[26]. Their contemporary, Pliny, reported that blood was used in the treatment of epilepsy, and Tertullian later wrote:

> 'Consider those who with greedy thirst, at a show in the arena, take the fresh blood of wicked criminals ... and carry it off to heal their epilepsy ... [Christians] do not even have the blood of animals at their meals ... At the trials of Christians you offer them sausages filled with blood. You are convinced, of course, that it is unlawful for them.'

The book *Flesh and Blood* reported that blood did not go out of fashion with the end of the Roman Empire: 'In 1483, for example, Louis XI of France was dying. Every day he grew worse, and the medicines profited him nothing, though of a strange character; for he vehemently hoped to recover by the human blood which he took and swallowed from certain children.'

By Louis's time, experiments with transfusing blood were all the rage, with just a few dissenting voices, like that of Thomas Bartolin, professor of anatomy at the University of Copenhagen, who objected strongly:

> Those who drag in the use of human blood for internal remedies of diseases appear to misuse it and to sin gravely. Cannibals are condemned. Why do we not abhor those who stain their gullet with human blood? Similar is the receiving of alien blood from a cut vein, either through the mouth or by instruments of transfusion. The authors of this operation are held in terror by the divine law, by which the eating of blood is prohibited. Either manner of taking it accords with one and the same purpose, that by this blood a sick body may be nourished and restored.

Joseph Priestley, who was a scientist and a clergyman – he invented soda water, too – shared this view of blood on theological grounds:

> 'The prohibition to eat blood, given to Noah, seems to be obligatory on all his posterity ... If we interpret the prohibition of the apostles by the practice of the primitive Christians, who can hardly be supposed not to

have rightly understood the nature and extent of it, we cannot but conclude, that it was intended to be absolute and perpetual; for blood was not eaten by any Christians for many centuries.'

Until the late seventeenth century blood was believed to be static in the body, subject only to tidal flows from time to time, so doctors concentrated on cleaning out the reservoir from time to time by way of sweating, vomiting, beating and purging the patient. In 1628 William Harvey had published his view that blood circulated in one direction only and then evaporated its way out of the body through tiny capillaries and pores in the skin, so that there was less need to top up the blood tank with transfusions, or to lower its levels with exfusions, or phlebotomy.

In the meantime, Real Medicine practitioners believed that it could easily become stagnant and need cleansing. Dr Willis, in a letter to his colleague Dr Hodge in 1670, suggested this prescription for purifying the blood, especially when plague was in the air[27]:

Electuary, Rx fresh flowers of borage, fumaria, white and red Lamia, of each 4 ounces.; pound well in a marble mortar; add 1½lb of white sugar, stirring it in and reducing it to a conserve. Add powder of red coral and ivory in a marble with juice of oranges, of each ½ an ounce, with similar quantities of syrup of coral. Make an electuary.

Powdered ivory and coral were in everybody's medicine chests for centuries, at least in part because they were expensive, inert, non-addictive and non-life threatening: whether they did any positive good was another matter.

For all our modern knowledge[28] of perils of whole-blood transfusions and the immune system, and with millions already infected with AIDS, as recently as 1991 some hospitals were still giving homologous blood transfusions as a tonic to anaemic patients, as they have been doing on and off since Giovanni Colle tried it in Italy in 1628 with largely tragic effect. It was only after Karl Landsteiner discovered the four principal blood groups in 1900 that patients started surviving transfusions and the number of fatal hemolytic reactions tailed off. When Pope John Paul was shot by a would-be assassin, he recovered quickly from the gunshot wounds, but was taken back to hospital for two months suffering from a cytomegalovirus infection that he had picked up from a blood transfusion.

An interesting fact about blood that you can introduce into any informal conversation is that the Incas practised blood transfusions on each other for some centuries with few fatal reactions, mainly

because all South American Indians are of the one blood group –
O-Rh-positive[29]. This fact deserves to be more widely known.

An intriguing book by Dr Michel Gauquelin[30] twenty years ago,
pointed to perceived links between blood, our health and the climate.
He observed that:

> Blood pressure problems occur mainly in the winter months (October
> to March in Northern Hemisphere); calcium and phosphate in the
> blood is at its minimum in February and March, its maximum in
> August; bleeding after treatment with anti-coagulants was at its
> maximum in January and February, its minimum in July; total blood
> protein, albumin and haemoglobin were often higher in winter than in
> summer.

He also claimed that:

> Surgeons know that complications occur more frequently at certain
> times. There is always the risk of complications during an operation,
> but the greatest dangers are post-operative accidents such as sudden
> haemorrhage and cardiac embolization ... one anesthetist reports that
> there are some days when it is very difficult to anesthetize patients and
> when patients stay in a disturbed state of post-anesthetic
> restlessness.[31]

Bones in the Throat

The Saxons ate a lot of meat, but lacked some of the finer points of
table etiquette. As a result bones, probably complete boars' ribcages,
lodged in their throats, but this was nothing to worry about for Saxon
technology could cope: 'To remove a bone sticking in the throat.
Take hold of the patient's larynx and say: "Blasius the martyr,
servant of God, saith, Go up, bone! or go down!" '

The alternative remedy from the Anglo-Saxon Leech Book,
though unlikely to win its author a prize for Scriptural knowledge,
was promised to work: 'Look at the patient and say: "Come up,
bone! whether bone or fruit, or whatever else it is; as Jesus Christ
raised Lazarus from the tomb, and Jonah out of the whale." '

Botts, the

This form of colic was generally believed to be caused by the botfly,
and may even have been linked to food poisoning (Latin *botulus*, a
sausage). The traditional treatment from the days of Galen onwards
was gentian (*Gentiana lutea*), a bitter preparation commonly used for
dyspepsia.

Breast, Inflammation of the

Wheezy chests are always with us, and now cholera is making a
comeback. Will it reach here? If so, be sure to invest in a pair of

wellies: 'The colic, inflammation of the breast and bowels, the iliac passion, cholera morbus, &c are often occasioned by wet feet.'

Breasts, Flagging
The herbal approach of Culpeper to this emblematic condition used the scatter-gun rather than the rifle, the shopping basket rather than the laser, with these multi-sourced rubs: 'Agrimony, Balm, Comfrey, Cross-Wort, Fig-Wort, Fleur-de-Lys, Groundsel, Hyssop, Mallows (marsh), Mint (garden), Mustard (hedge) and Plantain.'

But he also drew to our attention in 1675 the little-known gynaecological fact that heavy periods are caused by the breasts, and that rubbing them with celandines 'stayeth the overmuch flowing of the courses.' Male doctors were ever inclined to fantasize over the female body.

Broken Bones – see Fractures

Bubonic Plague, an Eye Witness Report
It takes an eyewitness report, in this case of Guy de Chauliac in 1348, to recall the horrors of septicaemic and pneumonic plague:

> The visitation came in two forms. The first lasted two months, manifesting itself as an intermittent fever accompanied by the spitting of blood, from which people usually died in three days. The second type lasted the remainder of the time, manifesting itself in high fever, abscesses and carbuncles, chiefly in the groin [buboes, hence 'bubonic']. People died from this in five days. So contagious was the disease, especially that with blood-spitting that no-one could approach or even see a patient without taking the disease. The father did not visit the son, nor the son the father. Charity was dead and hope abandoned.

The medical advice consisted of five simple steps:

1. Flee the region.
2. Purge yourself with aloes.
3. Exfuse a unit or two of blood.
4. Purge yourself with senna, had the fleeing not done so.
5. Cup and scarify the carbuncles.

Of these, (1) was undoubtedly the best advice, and (5) possibly the most tendentious, as poking about in infected buboes with an old knife was unlikely to do a lot of good.

Having fled, the recommended time to stay away was forty days, or in Italian, *quarantenaria*, from which we derive our word quarantine. The cause of the plague, incidentally, was: 'Eating garlic, pepper, and the meat of diseased hogs.' So it was all down to that number 54 with boiled rice, was it?

Burping, or Windiness

Embarrassment about burping, belching or otherwise discharging what the Americans call 'gas' has always been a nice little earner for the medical profession. It still is, with massive sales of patent medicines claiming to relieve the pressure, despite the cool advice of Joe Graedon, in his irreverent but scholarly work, *The People's Pharmacy*[32]:

> That's not to say it's impossible to have gas. Everyone does. It comes either from swallowing air while eating, or as a by-product of the digestion of food in the intestine. Gas is produced from the fermentation of undigested sugars, and some people have a harder time digesting certain foods, particularly beans, broccoli, onions and cabbage. Now hear this: Nothing – no OTC (Over The Counter) remedy – will alter the amount of gas your body produces. Gross though it may be, the only cure is to pass the gas.

He did suggest some ways of preventing the condition:

> First, please try to give up cigarettes. Stopping smoking is probably the best thing you could possibly do for your digestive tract. Losing weight can also be a big help, and if you can give up alcohol and aspirin, you would also be heading in the right direction. Fatty food, chocolate, coffee, orange juice, and spicy tomato drinks may also be adding to your woe.

As a pharmacist he urged readers against expensive seltzers and suggested instead half a teaspoonful of bicarbonate of soda in eight ounces of water – and not 'pigging out' on food.

Burping and Dr Foart Simmons

Two centuries ago a more adventurous view was taken. Dr Samuel Foart Simmons was looking for new medicinal uses for ether (*ethyl oxide*, the colourless, highly volatile product of heated sulphuric acid on alcohol): he had also become excited by laudanum, the liquid tincture of opium, these days containing 1 per cent of morphine and given in doses of five to thirty minims, but then largely home-made in varying strengths and dolloped out by the spoonful. Could they in any way be combined, he wondered?

Yes, they could: in his 1770 book he announced the thrilling news – some Real Medicine against gas was ready for the marketing department long before Joe Graedon was able to write his excellent book:

Mix a teaspoonful of aether, and a teaspoonful of laudanum, with a teaspoonful of peppermint water, and give it to the patient to drink as often as he can bear it.

The most common treatments are aether and laudanum with peppermint water, or opium in pills with asafoetida [a stinking gum from the roots of *Ferula foetida*, which was traditionally given as an anti-spasmodic for flatulence]. One teaspoonful to be taken with two teaspoonfuls of water, increasing the dose as much as the patient can bear it.

That prescription could well have ended in tears before bedtime. Indeed, in Dr Buchan's case notes there is a passing reference to a child thus treated by him in 1776. It was clinically successful. The lad even seemed to benefit for a day or two, but, the doctor added almost parenthetically, 'he was at length seized with a vomiting of blood, which soon put an end to his life'.

Elixir of vitriol (sulphuric acid in varying solution, mixed with cinnamon and ginger) was popular for a while. It was claimed to discharge wind, possibly through smoldering holes in the victim's body: 'From fifteen to thirty drops of elixir of vitriol, taken two or three times a day, will discharge wind and release the nervous system ... Aether, with a glass of French brandy wine, or ginger, are among the best medicines for expelling the wind.'

Or, for green prescribers seeking shrub-cred: 'Twelve to fifteen grains of rhubarb, half a drachm or two scruples of the Japonic confection, given every other evening, will have good effects.'

The herbalists' way of dealing with a burping client was typified by Nich. Culpeper's non-fatal recipe:

Take a pound of the wood and leaves of bitter-sweet [the woody nightshade, *Solanum Dulcamara*] together, bruise the wood, then put in a pot, and put to it three pints of wine; put on the pot lid and shut it close; and let it infuse hot over a gentle fire twelve hours, and then strain it out.

Take a quarter of a pint each morning. It purges the body very gently, and not churlishly as some hold. And when you find good by this, remember me.

Perhaps by placing a picture of him in your grateful loo.

Burping and the Vulgar, or 'Jasper', Carrot

The common, vulgar, or 'Jasper' carrot was supposed for centuries to cure burping, but Nicholas Culpeper was unsure whether Jaspers caused or broke wind:

Wild carrots belong to Mercury, and therefore break wind [only a
qualified astrologist could explain this use of 'therefore'] and remove
stitches in the side ... helpeth those whose bellies are swollen with
wind.

I suppose the seeds of them perform this better than the root: and
though Galen [Greek, 200-130 BC] commended garden carrots highly
to break wind, yet experience teacheth they breed it first, and we may
thank nature for expelling it, not they; the seeds of them expel wind
indeed, and so mend what the root marreth.

Caraway seeds crystallized in sugar served a similar purpose.

C

Cancer

Cancer has always been, and unfortunately still is, a terrible and
incurable disease, so it has afforded a fine field for all kinds of
nostrums and specifics all of which were promised to produce a 'safe
and certain cure'.

One of these from the sixteenth century, called 'precious water',
could have been composed in any home:

> Take dove's foote, a herb so named, Arkangell ivy with the berries,
> young red bryer toppes and leaves, whyte roses, with theyre leaves and
> buds, red sage, celandyne and woodbynde, of each lyke quantity, cut
> or chopped and put into cleane whyte wyne, and clarified honey. Then
> break into it alum glasse and put a little of the pouder of aloes
> hepatica. Destill these together softly in a limbecke of glasse or pure
> tin; if not then in a limbecke wherein aqua vitae is made. Keep this
> water close. It will not onely kyll the canker, if it be duly washed
> therewyth; but also two droppes dayly put into the eye wyll sharp the
> syght, and breake the pearle and spottes, specially if it be dropped in
> wyth a little fenell water, and close the eyes after.

By the 1770s the College of Physicians had reluctantly concluded
that cancer was 'incurable unless treated early'. Dr Buchan traced its
cause to 'eating farinaceous substances', thereby ruling out the
wholegrain bread, cereals and pasta that gained a magical status in

the self-obsessed eighties. The cures were external applications of nightshade, hemlock and – of course – mercury.

Cankers, or Small Ulcers
Mustard of the hedge (*Sisymbrium Officinale*) was recommended by Culpeper:

> It grows by the way and hedge-sides, and sometimes in open fields. It is common in the Isle of Ely. The juice, made into a syrup with honey and sugar, is effectual for coughs, wheezing and shortness of breath. The same is profitable for jaundice, pleurisy, pains in the back and sides, is used in clysters. The seed is good for ulcers and cankers in the mouth, throat, or behind the ears, and for hardness and swelling of the testicles, or of women's breasts.

Cataracts – See **Pin & Web**

Chancres
These lesions were very bad news, as their appearance frequently signalled the onset of syphilis. Dr John Hunter, whose work led to the founding of the Hunterian Museum, was interested in VD, even inoculating himself with Lues (q.v.) in the interests of research, but what thanks did he get? They named the hard chancre after him. Later, physicians jeered at him because he could not tell gonorrilis from syphilhoea. There was no cure.

Choler
A bitter humour (Greek *cholera*, bile) could produce a bitter and irascible character. No need for counselling or therapy, just shift the bile and the problem was solved. Herbalists for centuries up until the present time recommend asabaraca (hazelwort, *Asarum europaeum*), thyme, henbane or valerian (also still in use).

Cholera
Those who knew the cause could prescribe the cure: 'The colic, inflammation of the breast and bowels, the iliac passion, cholera morbus, &c are often occasioned by wet feet.'

Contemporary records give vivid descriptions[33] of this plague that once swept across Europe in tides of death. The first stage of the disease produced 'effortless and repeated diarrhoea without warning', described by any unlucky observers who had failed in their attempts to avoid being observers, as being 'like rice water.' Profuse vomiting followed.

The 'cold or choleric stage' followed, featuring collapse from loss of fluids, a rapid weak pulse, cold skin, severe thirst and cramps. In the 'febrile' stage the colour and pulse improved, giving relatives the impression that the sufferer was getting better, but death swiftly quashed these hopes.

Cholera – the York Plague

In the York plague of 1832, meticulously researched by Margaret Barnet[34], there were 450 cases recorded in a population of only 25,357, with 185 deaths. Her descriptions from contemporary records of the effects of mounting heaps of 'night soil' lightly covered with quicklime in slum streets with no drains or running water, provide a vivid picture of life in York and, presumably, other major cities of the time.

Doctors were clear about the treatment: Calomel [subchloride of mercury] every half-hour to control the secretions of the body; no liquids, just half a teaspoonful of water to help down the calomel. The shivering coldness could be controlled with mustard cataplasms [plasters] to stomach and limbs, heated sandbags and bricks. Mustard emetics would comfort the patient with a nice vomit. Five grams of ammonium carborate and same magnesium carborate went down a treat each half-hour with a glass of brandy.

If the patient was still alive, this was followed by the application of a few leeches, a blister, a blood exfusion of six to fourteen ounces taken from an arm, and more calomel every two hours.

Also tried in York was the cold water treatment to reduce the fever, as recommended by Dr Shute of Gloucester, but after two of a Dr Belcombe's patients died of it, the practice was grudgingly discontinued.

Dr Stevens' Saline Treatment, written up by the Royal College of Physicians two years earlier, proved to be less successful in the ward than it had been on the page, as is sometimes the case with learned papers. No one was cured, but neither was anyone killed by it, so it ended as a scoreless draw.

Dr Lawrie of Glasgow suggested cholera cases be given injections of laudanum and small quantities of whisky, and the patients, who were going to die anyway, were willing to give it a go. Others suggested transfusions of bullocks' blood or human serum – and they were all successful, except in that the ungrateful patients died.

Dr Needham of Goodram Gate used precise intravenous transfusions of: 'Two drachms of muriate of soda, two scruples of carbonate of soda, in 60 oz of water at 108-110F, injected by a Read's common syringe, to replace lost body fluids rapidly.' He experimented on thirty cases ('people' in lay language), only twenty-six of whom died[35].

All infected garments were 'removed with a pair of tongs' (try it on a friend tonight) and thoroughly boiled; other items were fumigated in sulphur for twenty-four hours.

Mr Culpeper had nothing interesting to say about cholera in his *Pharmacopoeia Londinensis*, or *London Dispensatory* of 1654, as the disease had not then been imported to Britain from India and Pakistan through Sunderland.

Clysters

Should you think that Clyster is a pretty name for a pretty girl in a pretty cottage, think again: a clyster was an enema. Dr Buchan found that it was easier to give clysters to children than nasty medicines that had to be spooned down recalcitrant throats:

> Wine whey is a very proper drink for children in an ague; to half an English pint may be put a teaspoonful of the spirit of hartshorn.[1] To children, it may be given as a clyster with half an ounce of extract of bark, dissolved in four ounces of warm water, with the addition of half an ounce of sweet oil [sulphuric acid], and fix with eight drops of laudanum [opium], given every fourth hour.

Hartshorn is generally described as a solution of ammonia in water, but Dr Buchan defines it as the horn of the red deer, rasped and boiled in water until it forms a jelly, to be used as a decoction. Wine whey was a very effective way of keeping children quiet, but it might have had one or two side-effects over the longer run, if there was one.

Cold Grief of the Mother

A mother's life was full of grief enough, one imagines, with earnest gynaecologists attacking her with every tool and product they could find, so if on top of that she were to suffer from long aching pains, she would be pleased to know that her husband had set some caraway (*Carum Carui*) in the garden, for

> Carraway seed hath a moderate sharp quality, whereby it breaketh wind and provoketh urine, which also the herb doth. The root is better food than the parsnips; it is pleasant and comfortable to the stomach, and helpeth digestion. The seed is conducing to all cold griefs of the head and stomach, bowels, or mother, as well as the wind in them.

If the pain persisted, she could always reach for the frying pan and the caraway plant: 'The herb itself, or with some of the seed bruised and fried, laid hot in a bag or double cloth to the lower parts of the belly, easeth the pain.'

Colic, or Cholic; also Lax and Continual Fluxes

Nicholas Culpeper took colic seriously in his *Complete Herbal* of 1645: your local police might take an equally serious view of anyone promoting it today:

Hemp (*Cannabis Sativa*) is a plant of Saturn. It is cultivated in many counties. It is sown at the end of March, or beginning April; and it is ripe in August or September.

The emulsion or decoction of the seed stays the lax and continual fluxes, eases the colic, and allays the troublesome humours of the bowels [known these days as 'alternative comedy'], it also stays bleeding at the mouth, nose, and other places.

There was a downside to the use of cannabis: 'Too much use of it dries up the seed for procreation.'

Culpeper might suggest that you accompanied your cannabis and opium with a tot of gin, for juniper berries also cured colic, and almost everything else – even orthopaedic problems:

There is no better remedy for wind in any part of the body, or the colic, than the chymical oil drawn from the [*Juniperis Communis*] berries. They are good for the cough, shortness of breath, consumption, pains on the belly, ruptures, cramps, convulsions, and speedy delivery to pregnant women; they strengthen the brain, fortify the sight, and strengthen the limbs of the body ... they stay all fluxes, help the haemorrhoids or piles, and kill worms in children.

How strange that juniper berries cured so many diseases in those days, and hardly any now. What has changed? Us, or the berries?

Colic, Windy
Windy people who had never comforted their lower belly with a fried caraway seed poultice during a colic attack were ready to forgive Mr Culpeper's enthusiastically random syntax and try that experience:

The roots of caraways eaten as men eat parsnips, strengthen the stomachs of old people exceedingly, and they need not to make a whole meal of them neither, and are fit to be planted in every garden. The herb itself, or with some of the seed bruised and fried, laid hot in a bag or double cloth to the lower parts of the belly, easeth the pains of the windy colic.

Common Cold, Preventing Without Drugs
John B. Keane, the sage of Listowel, recommends this ancient rural preventative for all colds[36]:

Soft, moist and greasy feet are to the rest of the body what sinfulness is to the soul ... it is to the dry foot that we must look if we are to expect our bodies as a whole to be healthy, which brings us back to last November and to this man I chanced to meet in the residents' lounge of a well known Cork hotel.
'I never get colds,' said he.

'I'm a martyr to colds,' said I.

'That's because you don't wash your feet,' said he.

'But I do wash my feet,' I replied without petulance.

'Of course you do,' said he, 'and so does every mother's son, but do you wash your feet every day?'

I shook my head.

'I wash my feet every day,' said he, 'and then I pull on fresh socks and dry shoes. Sometimes if the weather is particularly wet I wash my feet twice a day and pull on fresh socks twice a day and fresh shoes. You see, I never throw shoes away.

He wasn't in the least smug. He didn't have a cold. In fact he looked extremely healthy despite the fact that he looked an octogenarian at least.

So now.

Coughs, Both Chin & Chest

When a patient presented with a cough, the doctor had to decide whether it was a chin cough (whooping cough) or a chest cough (common or garden). For a chin cough they were likely to be given Decoction of Alcthen; this is how Dr Buchan prescribed it in 1776: 'Take of the roots of the marsh mallow moderately dried, three ounces; raisins of the sun, one ounce; water, three pints. Boil the ingredients in water till one third of it is consumed; then strain the decoction and let it stand for some time to settle. The decoction is used for an ordinary drink when coughing.'

For a rattling chest cough the prescription moved up a gear or two, with potentially addictive results: 'A mixture made of equal parts of lemon-juice, fine honey, and syrup of poppies, may likewise be used. Four ounces of each of these may be simmered together in a sauce-pan, over a gentle fire, and a tablespoonful of it taken at any time when the cough is troublesome.'

Coughs – Herbal & Other Opium Cures

Culpeper offered opium to his herbal fans, of course: '[Opium] incrassates thin serous acrid humours, and thus proves a speedy cure for catarrhs and tickling coughs.'

Angelica, Bilberries, Borage, Hazel Nut, Hemp (cannabis), Marsh Mallows, Black Mustard, Parsley, Parsnip, Rosemary and Sage were also cough cures, while onions were extra special: 'Being roasted under the embers, and eaten with honey, or sugar and oil, they much conduce to help an inveterate cough, and expectorate tough phlegm.'

Also, 'the gum of the cherry tree (*Prunus Cerasus*), dissolved in wine, is good for a cold or cough, and hoarseness of the throat.'

Courses, Bringing down Women's

Doctors who were puzzled by women's insides at least knew that

periods were meant to be regular; if they failed to be so, they had to
find ways of making them regular, even if it meant having to be cruel
(to the female patients) in order to be kind (to the husbands). The
Complete Herbal of 1654 took a kinder view ...

> 'Horehound [*Marubium Vulgare*] is found on waste dry grounds in
> England. It is a herb of Mercury. A decoction of the dried herb, with
> the seed, or the juice of the green herb taken in honey is a good remedy
> for a cough, or consumption. It is given to women to bring down their
> courses, to expel the afterbirth, and to them that have sore and long
> travails.'

Pennyroyal was another obstetric aid: 'Being boiled and drank, it
expelleth the dead child & afterbirth, & stayeth the disposition to
vomit.'

Cupping, Wet & Dry

Cupping was fun: they took a cup, burned some spirit in it, then
clapped it to a part of the punter's body, where the resulting vacuum
gave it a nasty suck and raised a weal. It was technical, expensive, of
no therapeutic value whatsoever and it hurt – so it 'worked'. For the
sceptical, the skin could first be scarified with a scalpel before
cupping, so that blood was sucked from the wounds; this was called
'wet cupping'.

It remained in the doctors' armoury until the 1970s and may still be
practised by present-day practitioners of Real Medicine in some parts
of the world.

D

Depression, not yet discovered, See Hypochondriac & Hysterical Complaints

Diagnosis, the Imperfect Art

Every physician was haunted by the fear that he would spot the
obvious – 'You've got a tickly ague' – and miss the less obvious – he
had been run over by a cart and lost both his legs. This worry was

exacerbated when the patient appeared to be a malingering hysteric, clamouring for medicines as children clamour for affection.

Dr Archibald Stevenson was practising in Edinburgh in 1699, and one of his regular customers was Lady Tarbett, whom he had down in his cryptic notes as a malingerer. In July Dr Stevenson wrote to Lord Drumcairnis with a letter, that was no doubt accompanied by his bill, explaining that there was nothing to worry about:

> Called be your sonne Mr. James to consult anent my lady's present state of health in the light of your lordship's letter and the information of some physicians with yow ... Wee did conclude that her ladyship's trouble is plainlie hysterick. I have seen my lady in many colicks and hysterick passions worse, according to information. I suggest strong purging and some of King Charles his famous Drops which are of the volatile spirit and spirit of raw silk. She should drink a posset made of sack and double-sweet milk of a cow.

While Dr Stevenson was out of town, no doubt seeing to another hypochondriac patient, his lordship consulted the doctor's partner, Dr Pitcairn, for a second opinion, as the lady did not seem to be improving. Dr Pitcairn loftily prescribed a 'simple' – what we would describe as some paracetemol – but dungier: 'My lord, if the pain continue in one place make a pultess of cow's dung, milk and camomil flowers and apply, or cause bake a bannock, let it be pease or bean meal, and Thiss apply warm to the places.'

The dung was no better than the posset, so Lord Drumcairnis consulted yet another specialist, Dr Pattison, on 8 August; he naturally pooh-pooed his colleagues' diagnoses and treatments as he offered his own solution to the lady's vapours:

> 'I have sent for my lady a great many of the anti-hysteric pills (within which is a verie small quantitie of opium well prepared). The King's Drops may be left off as they nauseate. The mixture ordered by your physicians there is proper enough against Vapours and may be taken by spoonfuls at any time her Ladyship is infected with a fit.'

Nobody seems to have discussed the nature of her illness with the lady herself; what sort of fits was she having? Was opium necessarily helpful? Was she just making it up? Possibly not, for on 9 October Provost Duff wrote to Lady Tarbett's husband a letter that was curt even by medical standards, claiming eight glasses of best whiskey as his fee for diagnosing what was by then wrong with her. She was dead. 'I knowed yesternight from Lord Tarbet shewing yt my lady's dead about twa oclock in the morning and withall I am about to send to you for eight balls of malt.'

It is the lack of humility that makes their errors seem so odd with

hindsight. In *Medical History*'s review of *Homeopathy in America* by
M. Kaufman, (1971, The Johns Hopkins Press) there is this cogent
point:

> Looking back one is inclined to smile at the spectacle of doctors,
> themselves groping around in the dark but not prepared to admit it,
> ready and anxious to accuse others of lacking in science, and it is hard
> not to look upon their postures and expostulations as a sign of their
> professional anxieties, jealousies and feelings of insecurity. What
> makes their behaviour the more discreditable is that the chief loser
> thereby was often the innocent patient.

Homeopaths were given a very rough ride by the medical
establishment, called 'allopaths' unless they practice in France, when
they are called 'allo-allo-paths.'

Diarrhoea
This was not a problem for doctors, as Dr Thornton pointed out in
1810: 'In diarrhoea, the disease itself generally carries off any
offending acrimony, and then opium is used with great effect.'

Diets or Regimens
Fashions come and go, but French chefs have never been happy to
share their skills with women. Bernard de Gordon encouraged male
chefs only to jolly up the invalids' diet in France in 1266: 'My own
opinion is that my master became ill through too much roast chicken
given him by women: but one cannot follow a decent diet when
women are in charge.'

John H. Appleby's commentary on John Grieve quotes the 1649
medical textbook *Regimen sanitatis Salerni* on dieting, with the
traditional emphasis on humours and astrology: '... in the time of Ver
or Spring, wee must eat little meat ... Red humours are increased and
specially flegmatick ... In Ver season, if one eat much meat, it lesseth
Nature to digest such flegmatick humours and causeth them to divert
one way or another way: For by those humours, and great quantity of
meat, Nature is oppressed. And so thereby such humours shall
remain in the body undigested, and run to some member, and there
breed some disease: and therefore we ought to take good heed, that
we eat not any grat quantity of meat in Ver.'

A doctor's job then was to create anxiety, especially about what
people ate, and it has never been difficult to do this.

Dr Samuel Foart Simmons, wrote against the evils of dairy produce
in 1780: 'Butter relaxes the stomach, and produces gross humours.'

In general, however, the eighteenth century put diet ahead of pills:
'A proper regimen, in most diseases, is at least equal to medicine,

and in many of them is greatly superior. Therefore the provision of proper food, fresh air, cleanliness, and other pieces of regimen are necessary in diseases, and is productive of many happy consequences.'

Encouragingly, wholemeal bread was suspect, even then.

Diet – Danger of Windy Bread
Fashions, as we have observed, change; two hundred years ago it was generally agreed that a high-fibre diet was ruinous to the health and contributed indirectly to global warming: 'Labourers generally eat unfermented bread, made of peas, beans, rye, and other windy things. They also devour great quantities of unripe fruits, baked, stewed, or raw, to fill the bowels with wind, and occasion diseases of those parts.'

No wonder that John Wesley had to carry his message of fresh food, fresh air and cleanliness to Britain in the face of considerable persecution. This from his 1782 sermon on dress: 'Let it be observed, that slovenliness is no part of religion; that neither this [1 Peter 3:3], nor any other text of Scripture, condemns neatness of apparel. Certainly this is a duty, not a sin. "Cleanliness is, indeed, next to godliness." '

Diphtheria – see **Measles**

Doctors
The structure of the medical profession from medieval times was much the same as it is today. There were, and arguably still are, three main branches to the profession:
plant doctors – today's prescribing practitioners
magic spell doctors – our psychiatrists and alternative therapists
saw-and-knife doctors – our surgeons
The specialisms were somewhat similar, too:

Proto-Homeopathy, developing from the assumption that like cures like – '*Similia similibus curantur*' – so eating foxes' lungs should, with a bit of luck, alleviate the distress of bronchitis, and a plant that looked like an ear should, if there were any justice in this world, cure deafness. It took a trained eye to spot the similarity between, say, a knee and a ragwort, but that was what made it all so fascinating. Today's homoeopathists have moved on from the mere visual similarity – the doctrine of signatures – to a more clinical approach.
Herbal Treatments, based on experimentation and experience gained over the millennia. Many of these treatments survive to this day, and feature in processed and concentrated forms in the British Pharmacopoeia. Some herbalists would say that processing and

concentrating herbs vitiates rather than consolidates their benefits. *Psychosomatic, or Unsympathethic, Medicine*, seeming to work by making the treatment worse than the disease. A child whose sore throat kept him in bed all day should recover quite quickly when offered live spiders to swallow whole. The sheer rigour of some early treatments suggests a desire to get people out of their beds and back to work – compare the design of Out Patients reception areas in many hospitals, making putative patients wonder whether being alive is all it is cracked up to be, or whether it might be better to crawl out into the car park and quietly die. If they can get into the car park.

Common Sense, like the thirteenth-century medical book that convincingly reasoned that a fracture patient should have a hole made in his bed 'so that he can relieve himself, otherwise it might be dangerous if he had to lie there forty days or more.' Or Dr Wesley's homely but novel advice to open cottage windows in fine weather and to drink clean rather than dirty water. Or Dr Simmons' advice in 1780 to avoid sunburn by eschewing excessive 'fleeping in the fun.' No sense is so common that it is not worth while repeating it out loud from time to time.

Doctors and Contracts

Doctors never quite knew where they stood socially. On the one hand, they were educated and highly paid men. On the other hand, they were indisputably in trade, and in mucky trade at that. At one time in the eighteenth century the doctor was so associated with trade that political cartoonists with the level of imagination that one sees in 'Spitting Image' were able to wax droll when a doctor's son became Prime Minister.[44] Henry Addington, later Lord Sidmouth, cringed when the public prints pointed out that '...for a Prime Minister to be a doctor's son was considered not only socially distressing but irrepressibly comical as well.'

Early in 1656, a Mr Stuteville wrote an admonitory letter to Sir Justinian Isham[45] about the dangers of the gentry's interbreeding with the mongrel breed of doctors:

> In these degenerating times, the gentry had need to be close neerer together, and make a banke and bulwarke against a Sea of Democracy which is over running them: and to keep their descendants pure and untainted from that mungrill breed, which would faigne mix with them ...
> I know a gentleman related to your Selfe, but a younger Brother and every way farre your inferior, who was offrd a very considerable fortune with a wife, beyond either his desert or expectation: yet because it was with a Physitian's daughter, the very thought of ye Blister-pipes did Nauseate his Stomacke. And great is the discourse at this very time about a Norfolk Baronets matching with a Doctor of

Divinities daughter in Cambridge, and yet we know that Divinitie is the highest, as Physicke is the lowest of professions.

Or there was John Lyly's 'Advice to gentlemen': 'Let thy practise be lawe, for the practise of physicke is too base for so fyne a stomacke as thine.'

The pay was always good, of course. The usual procedure was to charge a means-tested fee based on the value of the patient's house, like this mid-eighteenth century broadsheet:

RENTALS

	£10 to £25	£25 to £50	£50 to £100
Ordinary visit	2s 6d – 3s 6d	3s 6d – 5s	5s – 7s 6d
Night visit	Double an	Ordinary	Visit
Mileage beyond two miles from home	1s 6d	2s	2s 6d
Detention per hour	2s 6d – 3s 6d	3s 6d – 5s	5s – 7s 6d
Letters of Advice	Same charge	as for an	Ordinary Visit
Attendance on Servants	2s 6d	2s 6d – 3s 6d	3s 6d – 5s
Midwifery	21s	21s – 30s	42s – 105s
CONSULTANTS			
Advice or visit alone	21s	21s	21s
Advice or visit with another Practitioner	21s	21s – 42s	21s – 42s
Mileage beyond two miles from home	10s 6d	10s 6d	10s 6d

'Special visits i.e., of which due notice has not been given before the practitioner starts on his daily round, are charged at the rate of a visit and a half. Patients calling on the doctor are charged at the same rate as if visited by him.'

Despite the uncertain social status of doctors and surgeons, there were 32,000 of them at the time, serving a population of about 36,000,000 or one physician to 1,600 potential patients.

There are still occasional misunderstandings between GPs and the various health authorities, local or governmental, not about their social status, but rather about what is expected of them in return for their pay. This is partly because the role model that doctors have in their mind is an amalgam of all that was best in Dr Kildare, Dr Cameron and Dr Finlay.

The officials, however, have as their pin-up Dr Albrech von Haller (1708-1777), the Swiss-born average workaday GP who, according to *A Pictorial History of Medicine*, always managed to keep busy between house calls and surgery with a variety of laudable hobbies:

He produced a Chaldean grammar, a Greek and a Hebrew dictionary;
He wrote biographies and poetry and was an eminent novelist;
He taught all branches of medicine at Gottingen University and was a prominent anatomist, specializing in the physiology of blood vessels, the myogenic theory of the heartbeat and the role of bile in digesting fat;
He pioneered the study of angiology and microscopic anatomy;
He established botanical gardens;
He wrote thousands of scientific papers;
He was a prominent public health official;
He founded a refuge for orphans;
He was mayor of his local canton;
He wrote 14,000 letters to prominent figures of his day, many of which have by now been delivered; and, significantly,
He was never spotted anywhere near a golf course.

This is the standard to aim at if GP's want the administrators to warm to them, but even if they reach it they should still consider doing something useful on their half-day off each month, perhaps hosting a soirée for complainants and hypochondriacs.

Dr Buchan was in favour of informed consent and doctor-patient communication back in the 1770s, seeing in it a defence for both the profession and the public against the grosser abuses to which the system was susceptible: 'All we plead for is, that men of sense and learning should be so far acquainted with the general principles of Medicine as to be in a condition to derive from it some of those advantages with which it is fraught; and at the same time to guard themselves against the destructive influences of Ignorance, Super- stition and Quackery.'

Some early doctors assumed consent by demonstrating their gifts to their employers in an inappropriate manner, such that their appointments were immediately regretted. In the late eighteenth century Empress Maria Theresa appointed Lazzaro Spallanzani to the chair of natural history at Pavia University, and must have regretted her choice when he thanked her by swallowing cloth bags containing food, obtained gastric juices by vomiting them up again and demonstrated their ability to dissolve food in a test tube. She walked stiffly from the room and declined lunch.

The Chinese had three-level health care:

The superior doctor prevents disease,
The mediocre doctor attends to impending disease,
The inferior doctor treats actual sickness.

The less than inferior doctor can always write medical text books, possibly following some sound advice from Dr Richard Mead in 1812.[46]

> Should you have an itching to make your name known by writing a book on physic, I will advise you to choose a subject by which you will get most money; or that will bring you the most general business, as fevers, smallpox, etc ... The method of writing, if in your frontispiece you address not your book to some great man, is to club together with some other physicians; and thus by way of letters commend each other's good practice, and to support and to make each other favour. But above all things, take particular care, let the subject be what it will, that the words be well chosen, so as to make up an elegant and fervid speech; since you have ten to one [readers] that mind the language more than the ideas.

With advice like that many a doctor has found a second career in television, from interviewee to director general.

From the patient's point of view, the main object of the relationship was to see the doctor as rarely as possible and the surgeon never. Keeping out of harm's way has always been a laudable medical strategy, as this teaching of William Cullen, Professor of Edinburgh Medical School in 1770, showed:

> The preservation and healthful state of the body seems to be the objects which nature first recommends to the care of every individual. The appetites of hunger and thirst, the agreeable or disagreeable sensations of pleasure and pain, of heat and cold, etc. may be considered as lessons delivered by the voice of Nature herself, directing him what he ought to chuse, and what he ought to avoid, for this purpose ... Their principal object is to teach him how to keep out of harm's way.[47]

Doses, How to Tell Your Drachms from Your Scruples

Some units of measurement were hit-and-miss affairs: the quantity in a 'drop' would depend on the size of the aperture from which it dropped. Pills were made by rolling the mixture into a thin roll and cutting it into pieces for moulding into balls, with 'end pills' often being smaller than 'middle pills.'

Children's doses were in theory worked out by age rather than body weight, but cutting a pill into twelfths for an infant must have been problematic:

A patient between 20 and 14 may take ⅔ of the dose ordered for an adult
from 14 to 9, one half
from 9 to 6, one third
from 6 to 4, one tenth
and below four, one twelfth

Other units were more precise in 1771:

1 pound = 12 ounces	1 ounce = 8 drachms
1 drachm = 3 scruples	1 scruple = 20 grains
1 grain was the weight of a grain of dried wheat.	

The liquid measure was:

1 gallon = 8 pints	1 pint = 16 ounces
1 ounce = 8 drachms	

The 'cocktail effect' caused by taking a variety of medicines is not entirely understood. Joe Graedon in his *The People's Pharmacy*[48] gave specific deadly examples. Dr Buchan gave a similar warning two hundred years ago: 'Mixing the ingredients of a medicine, not only renders it more expensive, but also less certain, both in its dose and in its operation.'

Dover's Powders

It is impossible to read any old medical papers without finding references to these ubiquitous powders. They were named after their inventor, the doctor, privateer, South Seas entrepreneur and sometime charlatan, Dr Thomas Dover, of Bristow (Bristol) and Bath, according to Medical History's 1974 study, 'Dr Thomas Dover and the South Sea Company.' He was also the author of a bestselling medical book *The ancient physician's legacy*. His powders were a major success when made to his own recipe:

> Take Opium one ounce, Salt-Petre and Tartar vitriolated each four ounces, Ipecacuanha one ounce, Liquorish one ounce. Put the Salt-Petre and Tarta into a red hot mortar, stirring them with a spoon until they have done flaming. Then powder them very fine; after that slice in your opium, grind them to a powder, and then mix the other powders with these. Dose from forty to seventy grains in a glass of white wine Posset going to bed; covering up warm and drinking a quart or three pints of the Posset. Drink while sweating.

What did they 'cure'? Like all the best patent medicines, they were advertised as being 'good for what ails you'.

Dropsy, or Hydropic Disease

Although no longer regarded as a disease, but as a series of symptoms from disparate causes, dropsy used to be a big earner for all the competing branches of Real Medicine. Herbalists would reach first for the minty Pennyroyal, but Culpeper's vaunting claim for pellitory has the ring of confidence: 'If ever they have the dropsy, let them come to me and I will cure them gratis, using Pellitory of the Wall [poss. yarrow or feverfew; ME *peletre* from L *pyrethrum*, a sort of chrysanthemum or camomile, a known febrifuge]. It cureth also poor fickly neighbours.'

Should pellitory be out of season, there was always one of the herbalist's cure-alls – garlic: 'It is very useful in obstructions of the kidneys, and dropsies, especially in that which is called anasarca. It may be taken in a morning fasting, or else the conserve of Garlic which is kept in the shops may be used. It is held good in all hydropic diseases.'

But what springs to mind when Spanish Fly is mentioned? Exactly – dropsy and paralysis. Dr Brisbane in 1772[49]: 'A cry was raised in this capital against the internal use of cantharides, and the prejudice still remains in the minds of many physicians. By seeing the action of these insects on the skin and urinary passages when applied externally, it was natural to view them as poisons and a caustic.'

Since their dried bodies were useful externally as a counter-irritant, he judged them as good when taken internally for 'Paralytic affections, dropsies, stoppage of urine, asthmatic cases, some of which were very longstanding, and in hysterical disorders.'

Drunkenness

What caused drunkenness? Clearly it was not drinking too much, or doctors would not have prescribed such vast quantities of brandy, wine and beer. Could electrical fluid be involved in any way?

According to *L'Ésprit des Journeaux* in 1783, drunks were made such by the positive charge from the electric fluid in their booze. So a Dutch apothecary in Amsterdam suggested electrifying drunks with a negative charge to sober them up[50]. It seemed to work at the time.

Dumb Palsy, the

When Dr Johnson had his stroke, he lost his power of speech but not his gift of writing, nor his clear ideas on how he should be treated, as he showed in his letter to a friend, seeking Dr Heberdon's assistance in 1783:

> Dear Sir, It has pleased GOD, by a paralytic stroke in the night to deprive me of speech. I am very desirous of Dr Heberdon's assistance, as I think my case is not past remedy ...
> I think that by a speedy application of stimulants much may be done. I question if a vomit, vigorous and rough, would not rouse the organs of speech to action. As it is too early to send, I will try to recollect what

I can, that can be suspected of having brought this dreadful distress on.

I have been accustomed to bleed frequently for an asthmatic complaint; but have foreborne for some time on Dr Pepys's persuasion [Sir Lucas Pepys, Physician to King George III], who perceived my legs beginning to swell. I sometimes alleviate a painful, or more properly an oppressive, constriction of my chest by opiates; and have lately taken opium frequently, but the last, or two last times, in smaller quantities. My largest dose is three grains, and last night I took two. You will suggest these things to Dr Hemerdon.

Dysentery, When Travelling to Australia

In 1790 John White, Surgeon-General to the Fleet, published 'A Journal of a Voyage to New South Wales' (reported by Sir Edward Ford in his *Some Early Australian Medical Publications*) in which he reported on some new medical discoveries among the flora of Australia. Among them were astringent resins from the grass-tree (*Xanthorroea spp.*) and the red mahogany (*E. resinifera*); this was a major block-up of what had previously been a major breakthrough, and made life on board ship more bearable. Along with his innovative treatment of crew and convicts, involving fresh air, sanitation and regular exercise, he virtually removed dysentery from the list of shipboard miseries.

Another Australian discovery of his was the native eucalyptus tree whose distilled oil was of higher quality than that derived from the English *Oleum Menthae Peritae*. When Dr White sent a quart of eucalyptus oil to London it was New South Wales's first ever export of a domestic product.

E

Earth Bathing

Baron von Swieten's mid-eighteenth-century *Commentaries on Bocraeve*, was an interesting treatise on the health fashions open to the well-to-do of that day and among them was a fascinating vogue in Spain that seems about due for a revival at Balneologic Health Centres:

> In some parts of Spain, especially in Granada and Andalusia, they have a method of treatment by the use of an earth bath. Solano of

Luque advocated the 'baños de tierra', in which the patient was buried up to the chin in soil where no plant had grown, and left as long as he could bear. Solano would feed him meanwhile, and damp his temples. He would then be disinterred, wrapped in a linen cloth, and two hours later his whole body would be rubbed with an emollient ointment of leaves of solanum nigrum and hogs' lard.

Each time the patient was treated, a new pit had to be dug, since no pit was used twice. The best times for treatment were between early May and the end of October.

One young man of thirty years was thus interred, but had to be taken out after twenty minutes with an hysteric ague. He was later replaced in the loam, and endured this time an half hour, and was then rubbed with emollient ointments. In all he was buried five times, but having conceived a dislike to the process, he refused to submit to any further trials and died some months afterwards.

Electric Shock Treatment

Once electricity was discovered it was inevitable that some therapeutic function would be found for it. John H Appleby wrote a learned article on the pioneering work of John Grieve in the 1700s, work that placed him in that hazy hinterland of science where quacks and innovators were wont to meld.

Some Account of such Books and Discoveries as from their Novelty are become the objects of general Attention ... for the discoveries of Physickes, which have lately been announced to the Publick are many of them so extraordinary a kind, and hitherto so little ascertained, that I am often at a loss to judge whether they are fitter objects of belief or ridicule.

He put one part of oil of vitriol and two parts of water into a vessel into which he introduced an iron rod bent at right angles in such a Manner that one end remained in the fluid Mixture, while the other was applied to his Stomach [it might have been worse] – the consequence, he says, was that in about a quarter of an hour, he felt a heat which he qualifies with the words *douce et pénétrante*, diffuse itself over his whole body – this effect he attributes to the inflammable *gas* conveyed along the *iron*.

The second Experiment was with Electricity – on applying his hand to the back of the Person seated on the insulated chair the person felt the usual, prickling sensation, following the direction of the hand, which ever way it was moved; but on making the same movements with his hand after putting some crude Sulphur into the arms of his coat, the above Sensations increased in a very great proportion in so much so that several people by these means, from being cold, were made to sweat in the space of a few minutes [this was a Good Thing] – he calls this *Électricité Magnetizante* and proposes, to publish, in a short time some farther experiments with it.

Straightforward electric shocks were used to 'cure' epilepsy, toothache, hypochondria and whatever else ailed you, despite scientific evidence that it was useless. Why did the treatment survive the debunking? An article in *Medical History*[37] provides this interesting insight into the medical mind:

> ... the accumulated 'evidence' of the supposed influence of electricity on the body was too vast to be overthrown by the work of a single man, and most physicians in Holland and elsewhere blithely continued to use electricity as a major curative agent for many years to come ... [showing] the ease with which a subject can become acceptable, not because it has a strong theoretical background, but simply because a lot has been written about it.

Of course, all that has changed now. Definitely. Ask the marketing department of any pharmaceutical company.

Galvanism – early electric convulsive therapy – was also tried as a treatment for cholera in its second stage, together with rectal injections of 4oz to 6oz of turpentine. The knack was to keep any electric sparks well away from the treated area.

What gave them the idea that electricity had healing qualities? Priestley seems to have started it with his observation that it was because of the large amounts of electric fluid produced in certain animals such as cats and tigers that when they were highly aroused (i.e. when frightened or about to pounce on their prey) they gave off light[38]. Blake's little ditty did not help refute this theory of incandescent tigers.

Then a Dutch apothecary, Deiman[39], discovered in 1783 that Priestley's electric fluid only influenced the body when it could no longer pass freely through its pores and was therefore accumulated in the body or trapped outside, unable to get in. If the patient was insulated and then artificially electrified, the pulse rate and the rate of perspiration would increase until a stasis was achieved. Total poppycock (Dutch – soft excrement), but popular poppycock.

Another Dutch poppycocker, Boerhaave, saw the nerves as hollow tubes through which this liquid flowed, 'transmitting the orders of the soul to the body'.[40]

Haller, a Dutch scientist, calculated that this nerve-fluid travelled at 9,000 feet per second, and that the speed of the electrical matter was even greater. It could, he said, be used to treat various illnesses, including those caused by 'Paralysis; irregular workings of the principle of life; bad circulation of the fluids of the body; the prevention of the perspiration of body fluids.'[41]

English Physician Enlarged, the
It is easy to describe as seminal works that are subsequently seen as

having chuntered off down a cultural cul-de-sac, but few medical
works have had the impact or longevity of Culpeper's truly seminal
work, which is still being edited, altered and updated for reissue to a
believing public. An 1801 edition published in Berwick had this fly
leaf:

'The English Physician Enlarged
with Three Hundred & Sixty Nine
MEDICINES
made of
English Herbs
that were not in any IMPRESSION until THIS
being

An Astrologo-Physical discourse of the Vulgar Herbs of this Nation,
containing a complete Method of Physic, whereby a Man may preserve
his Body in Health, or cure himself, being Sick, for Three-Pence
Charge, with such Things only as grow in England, they being most for
English Bodies.
'Herein is also shewed these Seven Things, viz ... (2) What planet
governeth every Herb or Tree (used in Physic) that groweth in
England, (3) The time of gathering all herbs both Vulgarly and
Astrologically, (4) The way of drying and Keeping Herbs all the Year,
(5) The way of keeping their juice ready for Use at all times ... (7) The
way of mixing Medicines according to the Cause and Mixture of the
Disease and Part of the Body afflicted,

by Nich. Culpepper, Gent.
Student in Physic & Astrology.'

A twentieth-century edition removed all reference to astrology, which
was rather like reissuing the Bible for a post-Christian generation
without any reference to God:

'Culpeper's Complete Herbal –
consisting of
A Comprehensive Description of Nearly all Herbs
with their
Medicinal Properties
&
Directions for Compounding the Medicines
Extracted from Them.'[42]

Culpeper without the astrology has lasted a lot better than his
orthodox contemporaries with their dreadful specifics.

Epilepsy, or the Falling Sickness

The ancient writers were agreed: Aetius of Amida, Marcellus, Alexander Trallianus, all knew that carrying an amulet would solve the problem; the Leech Book of Bald gave the details: 'For onfall. Catch a fox, strike off the tusk from him while he is alive. Let the fox run away; bind the tooth in a fawn's skin; have it upon thee.'

Marcellus had only one cavill: he preferred to cut the tongue from a living fox and let it run – or crawl – away. Other Saxons believed it was the brain of the fox that protected children from epilepsy, but whether the fox ran away after its encephalotomy or not was never recorded, so there is no way of telling.

The author of the thirteenth-century medical textbook, *Practica*, had tried all that magic charm stuff and knew its limitations, which he set out in print: 'Let the reader note that I do not deal with certain affections, such as epilepsy, chronic toothache, paralysis, apoplexy, etc., because I think they are incurable.'

Mr Culpeper had no such doubts: one of his favourite remedies for absolutely everything including The Falling Sickness was All-heal or Woundwort [*Valeriana officinalis*]. Its rhizomes and roots, as you probably know, produce valerianic acid [$C_5H_{10}O_2$] in several isomers, as well as a volatile oil that is believed to act as a sedative on the nervous system, or, as they said in the seventeenth century: 'It kills the worms, helps the gout, cramp and convulsions, provokes urine, and helps all joint-aches. It helps all cold griefs of the head, the vertigo, falling sickness, and the lethargy.'

Cinquefoil (*potentilla* – five-leafed grass) also helped epileptics in their 'palsy': 'The juice hereof, drunk, with four ounces at a time, for certain days together, cureth the quinsy and yellow jaundice, and taken for 30 days together, the falling sickness.

'Wash your hands often herein and cures palsy – let it dry itself, do not wipe it off.'

Garlic, of course, was used, for 'This was anciently accounted the poor man's treacle [remedy], it being a remedy for all diseases and hurts.'

Back-up plants included Betony, Briory, Cowslips, Foxglove, Misselto and Saffron in various decoctions.

For those seeking a more radical cure, up at the sharp end of advancing technology, there were always skulls, according to Dr Camillo Brunoni in 1726:

Skulls of persons who have died a natural death, are good for little or nothing. The reason for this is, that the disease of which they died has consumed or dissipated the essential spirit. The skulls of murderers and bandits are particularly efficacious. And this is clearly because not only is the essential spirit of the cranium concentrated therein by the nature of their violent death, but also the force of it is increased by the long exposure to the atmosphere, occasioned by the heads of such persons being ordinarily placed on spikes over the gates of cities. Such skulls are used in various manners. Preparations of volatile salt, spirit, gelatine, essence, etc., are made from them, and they are very useful in epilepsy. The notion soldiers have, that drinking out of a skull renders them invulnerable in battle, is a mere superstition, though respectable writers do maintain that such a practice is a proved preventive against scrofula.

Euthanasia

In a sense, all medicine of this era was unintentional euthanasia. When the wandering surgeon Ambroise Paré reached Turin in 1580 he came upon three soldiers with gunshot wounds. His treatment of the wound was to pour on 'oil of elders scalding hot', but it did not help the men, who needed something more:

> They neither saw, heard, nor spoke, and their clothes were still smouldering with gunpowder. As I was looking at them with pity, there came an old soldier who asked me if there was any way to cure them. I said, No. Then he went up to them and cut their throats, gently and without illwill, so they 'would not linger in misery'.

Who did right? The old soldier or the surgeon?

Exercise, Folly of

Is exercise ever good for us? Dr Buchan thought it had its drawbacks: 'It is certain that too much exercise will prevent sleep.'[43]

French doctors in 1348 shared their British colleague's disapproval of sports shops and health food shops:

Do not sleep during the day.
Do not eat cold or moist food.
Do not go out at night.
The consumption of olive oil is fatal.
Bathing is dangerous.
Any exercise is dangerous.
Sexual indulgence is particularly dangerous.

What did that leave for people who wanted a fun time and did not even have the telly?

F

Falling of the Fundament

Whether it was the rectum or the womb that prolapsed, it was
obviously a good idea to rinse it and pop it back in place. Dr Willis, in
an undated letter some time in the mid-seventeenth century, went
further in suggesting this design for a patent rectal truss:

> The wastband is to goe about the middle, the points are to truss it up to
> your doublet. If you must weare it in the night, the claspholes are to
> bee fitted to claspes that are to bee on the skirts of the canvas
> waistcoat. But if you need it not in the night you may take all the eyes
> or the claspholes off. The button is to bere on the fundament to booy it
> up, and the bag is for the members, the two straps are to come up on
> each thigh, and the clasp holes to fit to the claspes on the wastband.

Felons

Culpeper knew how to treat troublesome sores on the fingers:
'Country people commonly use to take the berries of woody
nightshade [*Solanum Dulcamara*], and having bruised them, they
apply them to the felons, & thereby soon rid their fingers of such
troublesome guests.'

Fevers, Intermittent, Remittent, Inflammatory, Nervous, Purple, Yellow & Black

In 1776 doctors viewed the human body as an unclean receptacle full
of noxious substances, so if it overheated it was simply a sign that the
doctor needed to empty the dustbin and give it a good rinse: 'The first
thing to be done in the cure of an intermittent fever, is to cleanse the
stomach and the bowels. Vomits are to be administered before the
patient takes any other medicine; usually this will be a scruple of
ipecacuanha, or half that for a child.

In later editions, Dr Buchan got tougher with the fever with an
incredible series of blood exfusions: 'If after the first bleeding [12 – 14

ounces] the fever should increase, and the pulse become more frequent and hard, there will be a necessity for repeating it a second, and perhaps a third, or even a fourth time, which may be done at the distance of twelve, eighteen, or twenty-four hours, as the symptoms require.'

The various kinds of fevers all received the same treatment, but some took longer than others.

Fluxes of the Humours

It was no joke if your humours started fluxing, because they could make your eyes sore, according to Dr Buchan's fourteenth edition in 1794:

> Collyrium of alum: Take of alum, half a drachm; agitate it well together with the white of an egg. It allays heat and restrains the flux of the humours. It must be spread upon linen, and applied to the eyes.
>
> Collyrium of Lead. Take sugar of lead, and crude sal ammoniac, of each four grains. Dissolve them in eight ounces of common water; forty or fifty drops of laudanum may be added to this collyrium.

This latter collyrium more or less corresponds with Goulard's Water, popularly used in modern times on warm flannel for the treatment of sprains, bruises and inflammations, though not notably on sore eyes.

Foreign Travel, Perils of

Englishmen have always been appalled at the fact that so much of planet Earth is abroad. They tried to rectify the situation by turning a third of it into the British Empire, but its subjugated inhabitants remained irritatingly foreign. The Church of England's Recessional reflected this fearful contempt of foreigners with its talk of 'lesser breeds without the Law,' and doctors weighed in with equally fearful warnings of the dangers involved in foreign travel. Gilbert English, or Gilbertus Anglicus as he was known when on duty up the monastery, said this about going abroad back in the 12th century, long before air traffic controllers got into the habit of going on strike every peak holiday season:

> Before travelling across the sea I counsel a preliminary purgation, a good bath, ample meals to build up one's strength, electuaries to guard against the heat in summer, and heating electuaries to guard against the damp and misty air in winter.
>
> Every evening he should take a light supper, wash his feet in hot water and rub his soles with salt. On hot days he should keep his head covered, and quench his thirst with vinegar and water. Bread at least three days old should be preferred for meals, together with goat flesh,

pork, poultry, fish that have scales, but no milk products should be taken except in the evening.

Travellers on the old Swansea to Cork route will sympathise with sea travellers two hundred years ago:

> To prevent nausea and vomiting on ships, avoid foul smells. If he becomes seasick he should suck sour pomegranates and eat nothing until his stomach is settled.
> To overcome the stench of the ship, he should after each meal chew cloves of musk, or amber, and carry an amber apple in his hand, and put it to his nose. As far as is possible he should keep clear of the bilge channels by walking on the top deck. To avoid fleas and lice his clothes should be washed frequently. Drinking water should be strained, allowing the sediment to settle.

The latter injunction is becoming piquantly familiar to present-day users of profitized water.

In 1825[44] Dr Abernethy put the Royal College of Surgeon's view of Abroad in densest medical prose: 'Persons of particular constitutions are predisposed to those febrile actions of the sanguiferous system, which constitutes the inflammatory fever; there is a propensity to convulsions in children; & to tetanus in the inhabitants of warm climates.'

Historian D W Taylor recalled some manuscript lecture notes of Alexander Monro primus of 1725 that knocked on the head any idea of chilled wine beside the pool or cold lager on football's summer terraces:

> If after heating by exercise, or any other way would swallow down a quantity of any cold Liquor, or expose himself to a cold Wind, by the sudden Contraction from the cold of the Vessels, which were before very much dilated, he could hardly escape one of the Inflammatory Deseases, such as Angina, Pleuritis, etc, a Phlegmon, or Erysipelas externally.

Has the medical profession adjusted to the ordinariness of foreign travel in this sophisticated age of supersonic flight? Not really. They still cry havoc and let loose the dogs of war when anyone talks of venturing across the Channel. Dr Smith[45] listed these familiar perils of holidays and foreign travel in the 1980s:

> Sea sickness; diarrhoea; constipation; indigestion; headaches; extensive, deep burns; heat stroke; sunlight; sewage; drowning; dogs' mess; ice cream; insect bites; psychological trauma; jet lag; inner-ear infections; nausea; insomnia; dehydration, pulmonary embolism [from sitting too long on airline seats]; deep vein thrombosis; hepatitis B;

AIDS; typhoid; malaria; dysentery, contaminated blood transfusions; reckless driving; brandishing weapons at other drivers; shootings in cars, and near collapse.

Are the risks over-stated just a little? Ask any returning holidaymakers as they step off their chartered flight.

Fractures
A thirteenth-century medical book convincingly reasoned that a fracture patient should have a hole made in his bed 'so that he can relieve himself, otherwise it might be dangerous if he had to lie there forty days or more'. If asked, nurses would have suggested putting a container beneath the hole, but nobody asked.

Freckles & Spots
According to Nich. Culpeper, 'The meal of oats boiled with vinegar and applied, takes away freckles and spots in the face, and other parts of the body.' An alternative was the common onion: 'The juice is good. Used with vinegar it takes away all blemishes, spots, and marks in the skin. Applied also with figs beaten together, helps to ripen and break imposthumes, and other sores.'

Tougher abscesses called for tougher treatment using garlic: 'It is a good preservative against, and a remedy for, any plague, sore or foul ulcer; takes away spots and blemishes in the skin, eases pain in the ears, ripens and breaks imposthumes, or other swellings.'

French Pox, or Morbus Gallicus – see Venereal Disease

Ftupidnefs, including Dullness of Mind
It is difficult to guess what precisely doctors had in mind three hundred years ago when they spoke of 'stupidness' as a brief, curable condition. Rosemary helped the curative process, for, as Culpeper tactlessly pointed out, 'Rosemary is under the celestial ram': 'The decoction thereof in wine, helpeth the cold distillations of rheums into the eyes ... giddiness or swimmings in the head, drowsiness or dullness of the mind and sense like a ftupidnefs, the dumb palsy, or loss of speech, the lethargy and fudden fickness; to be both drank, and the temples bathed therewith.'

School teachers must be in the market for anything that can perform miracles of that order.

Fustigation
Country doctors carried a staff, often with a heavy metal head. Why was this? According to J.C. Jeaffreson's *Book about Doctors*, it was part of their therapeutic equipment: 'For many centuries fustigation

was believed in as a sovereign remedy for bodily ailments as well as moral failures, and a beating was prescribed for an ague as frequently as for picking and stealing.'

Fustigation was later replaced by 'rubbing the belly with brandy and salt' or drinking a suspended solution of opium and chalk. Perhaps during the overlap period they had a choice.

G

Gonorrhoea

The name illustrates the confusion about the disease, coming from the Greek for a flow or discharge of sperm, for which the mucus was mistaken. In any case, doctors and quacks of the seventeenth and eighteenth century reached for mercury, whether 'Crude, calcinated, Aethiop's minerals, calomel, corrosive sublimate, red precipitate, white precipitate.'

See also Venereal Disease

Gout

Gout was widely but wrongly believed to be a self-inflicted wound occasioned by consuming too much port and game, an indulgence which caused 'morbid humours' to 'drop' [Latin *gutta*, gout, a drop] onto joints. Galen of Pergamum, whose first-century medical writing influenced medical thought well into the Middle Ages, chimed with the received view when he described it as 'an unnatural accumulation of humours in a part' and blamed self-indulgence and luxury, as doctors have always tended to: 'This painful disease in a great measure proceeds from indigestion, and an obstructed perspiration.'

Dr Thomas Shorley, physician to Charles II, eschewed blame while his apprentices chewed bones:

> Calomel should be administered in simple doses. Sugar of lead be mixed largely in his conserves; pulverised human bones he was very fond of prescribing; and the principal ingredients of his gout-powder was raspings of a human skull unburied. But his sweetest compound was his Balsam of Bats, strongly recommended as an unguent for

hypochondriac persons, into which entered adders, bats, sucking-whelps, earth worms, hogs' grease, the marrow of a stag, and the thigh-bone of an ox.

Of these tasty ingredients the calomel and hogs' grease remained longest on the apothecaries' shelves, seeing service into the nineteenth century. The rest were consigned to gastronomy, where they became the basis of rural Hungarian goulash.

Meanwhile medical science marched on, seeking to outgrow its pervasive humorous view of illness. In The Sydenham Lecture given at the Apothecaries Hall in 1973, there was this reference to a possible cosmic cause of gout that had been identified by scientists in 1683, one that removed all blame from the sufferer and admitted rich food back onto the diet sheet:

> Whether the inward bowels of the earth undergo various changes by the vapours which exhale therefrom so that the air is tainted, or whether the atmosphere be changed by some alterations induced by some peculiar conjunction of any of the heavenly bodies, it is a truth that at particular times the air is stuffed full of particles which are hostile to the economy of the human body.
>
> At these times whenever we draw in with our breath such noxious and unnatural misasmata, mix them with our blood, and fall into such epidemic diseases as they are apt to engender, Nature calls in Fever as her usual instrument for expelling from the blood any hostile materials that may lurk in it.

Thus Thomas Sydenham had helped to shift causation of disease from the wrath of God, or an unfortunate alignment of the planets, to his 'morbific particles'. His discovery made everyone feel happier, because it is comforting to be told that one is not ill, but has a virus, or something is 'going round at the moment', or that a subterranean force has just belched up some morbific particles.

When Stephanie Blackden wrote an article on Samuel Johnson's gout[46], she quoted Sir John Hawkins' book, *The Life of Samuel Johnson* (Jonathan Cape 1962) on the great man's struggle for mobility: 'What a man am I, who have got the better of three diseases, the palsy, the gout, and the asthma, and can now enjoy the conversation of my friends, without the interruption of weakness or pain!'

Johnson's ode in *Gentleman's Magazine* 1747, written when he was 'ill of the gout' linked gout with arthritis, but doctors are no longer sure that his diagnosis was correct:

Unhappy! whom to beds of pain
Arthritick tyrannt consigns
Whom smiling nature courts in vain
Tho' rapture sings, and beauty shines.

Whether or not it was gout that struck him in his old age, he was able to write out a prescription for himself:

Besides my constant and radical disease, I have been these ten days much harassed with the gout, but that has now remitted ... I could not without many expedients and repeated efforts raise myself in my bed; nor without much pain and difficulty by the help of two sticks convey myself to a chair. Dr Brocklesby allowed large doses of opium which naturally eased the pain. It then withdrew in part from the right foot, but fell furiously upon the left. But I now walk alone.

What raises doubt about the diagnosis is the curious fact that so many people died of gout: in 1774, for instance, 54 out of 21,000 deaths in London caused by gout, or 2.5 per 1000, a figure that is implausibly high for this constitutional disorder. None of these doubts worried Sam Johnson as he snorted opium and tried to hide from Boswell.

Gout and the Gall of an Ox
The first recourse of the BUPA brigade was a trip to Bath and its magic waters, but the arthritic poor, living in Christina Rossettiesque villages far from private medical care, knew that gout-curing miracles were being worked for patients like themselves on a daily basis simply by strapping a piece of raw lean beef round the affected leg or foot, and changing it every twelve hours; or rubbing the parts with a raw onion. There was a vegetarian alternative, a poultice of warm honey, also changed every twelve hours. Or: 'An ointment made from mixing together the gall of an ox with a piece of fat chicken, rubbed in well, will stop the gout from getting worse.'

The fourteenth-century *Practica* had said with Harley Street hauteur that it was *'chacun a son gout'*: 'I have nothing useful to say [about gout], so I will not burden my pages with it, for I boldly assert that surgery and physic are useless, and I consider it incurable and unworthy of attention.

More positive souls, who thought their ague well worthy of attention, held that the poisonous lily of the valley possessed many healing qualities, though not under ordinary circumstances; it needed processing to get the best gout-quenching qualities out of it: 'If the flowers of the lily of the valley, closed up in a glass, are put into an ant hill, and taken away again a month later, ye shall find a liquor in the glass, which being outwardly applied, helps the gout.'

Gleet, see Venereal Diseases

Gravel
Small kidney stones caused acute pain and discomfort, but before asking the doctor for some mercury, or the surgeon for a bleed, some would have asked their local old wife for some ideas. She would have recommended drinking some water in which ripe hop heads had been boiled, perhaps with a little saffron to colour it, for this would 'cleanse the reins of gravel' without side effects.

Sometimes they took black cherries 'bruised with the stones and dissolved, the water thereof much used to break the stone and to expel gravel and wind'.

H

Hair, Promoting Growth of
Culpeper suggested gathering Cinquefoil (*Potentilla*), reducing it to a decoction (much the same as a *court-bouillon*) and rubbing it into the scalp. No guarantee, but it also cured agues 'in three fits'.

Hair, to Make Fashionably Yellow
A balm could be made, according to Culpeper, from mustard seed, ground into an emulsion and rubbed into the scalp; also provoked growth of hair with hardly any blistering or agony to speak of, really.

Hardness of the Breasts
Dr Thornton in 1810 suggested leaving the kitchen to nip down to the tobacconist for help with tumours on or near the breasts: 'Tobacco is sometimes used externally in unguents. Beaten into a mash with vinegar or brandy, it has sometimes proved serviceable for removing hard tumours from the hypochondres; an account is given in the Edinburgh Essays of two cases of the kind cured by it.'

Only two? That makes tobacco mash sound distinctly dodgy. In any case, the old herbal remedy of mustard seed mixed into a syrup with honey and sugar, or even mustard seed ground into an ointment, is probably safer for hard breasts. See also **Testicles, Hardness of.**

Heart Disease and Hemlock

Rumblings, murmurs or palpitations of the heart could be treated, but the causes could not, because no-one knew for sure how the heart worked or even what functions it performed:

> Take any quantity of the extract of hemlock [*Conium maculatum*], and adding about one fifth part of its weight of the powder of the dried leaves, form it into pills of the ordinary size. From one to several in the day, increasing the dose gradually, and as far as the patient can bear them, without any remarkable degree of stupor or giddiness.

This narcotic anti-spasmodic was alto used in those days against epilepsy and whooping cough, but not any longer.

Herbalism & Astrology

Although doctors studied botany along with chemistry and midwifery, they were often worried by herbalism's links with astrology. Culpeper's definitive work was astrological in essence, not just in detail, because the influence of the plants was crucial on the plant and even on the time of its picking, to the extent that a planet chart and calendar would have been the first items in such a doctor's black case. For example:

Table of all the Herbs in this Book; as to what PLANET governeth every one of them:

Adder's Tongue	is under	Moon in Cancer
Common alder tree	is under	Venus
Basil	is under	Mars in Scorpio
Eyebright	is under	the Sun in Leo

He also made inscrutable comments that would baffle many a pharmacist – or greengrocer – like:

> Lettuce – the moon owns it
> Pepper wort is a martial herb
> Solomon's Seal – Saturn owns the plant
> Wild Tansy – Venus rules it
> Our Lady's Thiftle is under Jupiter

Or this comment on woundwort, his all-purpose proto-antibiotic:

> Hercules learned its properties from Chiron. It is under the dominion of Mars, hot, biting and cholerick; & remedies what evils Mars afflicts the body of Man with, by sympathy, as the loadstone iron.
> It kills the worms, helps the gout, cramps and convulsions, provokes urine, and helps all joint-aches. It helps all cold griefs of the head, the vertigo, falling fickness, and the lethargy.

This combination of botanical fact with superstitious mumbo-jumbo always tended to keep the disciplines apart, like Culpeper's claims for Bitter-sweet, or woody nightshade (*Solanum Dulcamara*): 'It is under the planet Mercury and a notable herb of his also, if it be rightly gathered under his influence. Good also to remove witchcraft in men and beasts, as also all sudden diseases whatsoever. Being tied around the neck, it is one of the admirablest remedies for the vertigo or dizziness in the head that is.'

No wonder professional physicians had such an uneasy flirtation with ancient herbal remedies. Dr Robert Thornton sought, in 1814, to right the unprofessional wrongs perpetrated by medical outsiders like Culpeper, but the dedication of his book[47] was a classic banana skin just waiting for his neat Harley Street foot: 'The present Work, therefore, is presented to the world as a more complete and Perfect HERBAL than has hitherto appeared.[48]

> A desire to become acquainted with the virtues of Plants seems to have been coeval with the first dawn of knowledge; but the figures contained in the books treating of these subjects are so inaccurate, and the descriptions so vague, credulous, and, in every sense, so gross and vulgar, that mistakes were unavoidable, and false properties were bestowed on the most common and trivial Plants.

Blowing one's own trumpet while stepping on a banana skin is unwise. In this same perfect herbal pharmacopoeia, this more perfect doctor had this to say about the clinical uses of tobacco: 'Injections by the anus of the smoke or decoction of tobacco have been used with advantage in cases of obstinate constipation threatening ileus, of incarcerated hernia, of ascarides, of spasmodic asthma, and of persons apparently dead from drowning or other sudden causes.'

Gross and vulgar? From a man who habitually puffed tobacco smoke up the anus of any drowned man he came across? He was lucky there was no 'Carry On' team in those days to record his exploits on film.

Herniotomists – see **Barbers**

Hippocratic Oath
This oath had less to do with patient care than one might have imagined. Its first priorities, alas, were money and the closed shop and only then was patient care addressed, along with an extinguished promise not to perform abortions.

> I swear by Apollo Physician, by Asclepius, by Health, by Heal-all, and by all the gods and goddesses, making them witnesses, that I will carry out, according to my ability and judgment, this oath and this indenture: To regard my teacher in this art as equal to my parents; to make him partner in my livelihood, and when he is in need of money to share mine with him; to consider his offspring equal to my brothers; to teach them this art, if they require to learn it, without fee or indenture; and to impart precept, oral instruction, and all other learning, to my sons, to the sons of my teacher, and to pupils who have signed the indenture and sworn obedience to the physicians' Law, but to none other. I will use treatment to help the sick according to my ability and judgment, but I will never use it to injure or wrong them. I will not give poison to anyone though asked to do so, nor will I suggest such a plan. Similarly I will not give a pessary to a woman to cause abortion. But in purity and in holiness I will guard my life and my art. I will not use the knife on sufferers from stone, but I will give place to such as are craftsmen therein. Into whatsoever houses I shall enter, I will do so to help the sick, keeping myself free from all intentional wrongdoing and harm, especially from fornication with woman or man, bond or free. Whatsoever in the course of practice I see or hear (or even outside my practice in social intercourse) that ought never to be published abroad, I will not divulge, but consider such things to be holy secrets. Now if I keep this oath and break it not, may I enjoy honour, in my life and art, among men for all time; but if I transgress and forswear myself, may the opposite befall me.

Apothecaries or pharmacists, who for years were members of the Grocers' Company, had a far sterner set of requirements for apprentices to their trade, as this extract from the proceedings of the Scottish Society of the History of Medicine shows. A young man was signing his indentures as an apothecary and surgeon in February 1692:

> That is to say The said John Campbell by the tenor hereof becomes bound Apprentice and Servant to the said Adam Drummond in his Arts and Calling of Surgery and Pharmacy for all the days space years and Terms of five years next and immediately following his Entry thereto ...
> Obliges him to serve the said Adam Drummond his said Master faithfully and honestly by day and by night, Holy day and Work day in all things Godly and Honest; And shall not hear of his said Master's

skaith at any time by day or by night during the space forsaid, but shall reveal the same to him and hinder it to his power;

And that he shall not reveal his Master's Secrets in his Arts. Nor the Secret diseases of his patients to any person whatsoever; Nor shall be absent himself from his said Master's service at any time during the space forsaid without his Master's Special Licence had and obtained of him for that effect.

And that he shall not committ (as God forbid) the filthy crimes of Fornication or Adultery nor play at any Games whatsoever and that he shall not be Drunk, nor a Nightwalker, nor a haunter of debauched or Idle company; and that he shall not disobey his Masters Orders pretending he is Elder or Younger Apprentice, Or upon any other pretence whatsoever; and that he keep his ordinary Dyets at Bed and Board unless he is drawn into his Masters necessary affairs and Employment and no other ways: And that he shall not go any of the Professors of Medicine Chymie Anatomy Surgery or Materia Medica during the first three years of their Indentures ...

And that during the space of their Indentures he shall not be guilty of, nor accesory to the raising of any Tumults or Uproars within the town of Edinburgh or Suburbs thereof.

Hoarseness of the Throat

During the summer, amateur practitioners of Real Medicine could be seen scraping the bark from cherry trees (*Prunus Cerasus*) in much the same way as more serious people scraped the opium poppy. The old wives' fans knew that '... the gum of the tree dissolved in wine, is good for a cold cough, and hoarseness of the throat; it also mendeth the colour in the face, sharpeneth the eyesight, and provoketh the appetite.'

Now there is a spray that stops the healing gum from forming.

Hockogrockle, the see Quacks

Hypochondriac & Hysterical Complaints

Dr Hemerdon, who looked after His Majesty's illnesses at the eighteenth century's end, was a thoughtful man who pondered a question that did not seem to occur to many of his contemporaries: it was the problem of depression unrelated to observable morbidity:

Our great ignorance of the connexion and sympathies of body and mind, and also of the animal powers, which are exerted in a manner not to be explained by the common laws of inanimate matter, makes a great difficulty in the history of all distempers, and part of this. For hypochondriac and hysterical complaints seem to belong wholly to these unknown parts of the human composition; the body itself, as far as our senses are able to discern, seeming to have all its integrity and imperfection in those who have long and greatly suffered by these disorders. But there is hardly any part of the body which does not sometimes appear to be deeply injured by the influence of great dejection of spirits.

Where others prescribed alcohol, opium or cannabis, this good doctor tried to find both cause and cure in the patient's lifestyle.

Hysteric Fits, How to Handle a Woman

Hysteria (Greek – 'the old womb is playing her up again') was a frequent female condition, sometimes alleged to be linked to spirit possession, but every physician worth his mercury salts knew How to Handle a Woman:

A sudden suppression of the menses often gives rise to hysteric fits. These sometimes resemble a swoon with strong convulsions, immoderate fits of laughter, or crying.

It is customary during hysteric fits to bleed the patient. Rouse her by strong smells, as burnt feathers, asafoetida, or spirits of hartshorn [ammonia smelling salts] held to the nose. Hot bricks may be applied to the soles of her feet, and her belly may be strongly rubbed with a warm cloth. The best application is to put the feet and legs into warm water. Some cordial julep may be given, with opium, camphor and musk.

Blistering plasters applied to the part affected will often be sufficient to remove the complaint.

This technique, though thorough, carried no guarantees of success.

In earlier times hysteria was not a problem for doctors, as convulsions and hysteria were assumed to be the result of spirit possession,[49] but herbalists turned, as they very often did, to their favourite plant, now in the form of Pennyroyal Water: 'Take of pennyroyal leaves [*Mentha pulegium*, mint-scented], dried, one pound and a half; water, half a gallon to two gallons. Draw off by distillation one gallon. Give in drink as a julep to anxious or hysterical persons.'

I

Ileus, or Iliac Passion
An obstruction of the intestine, with intense pain and vomiting, was an interesting challenge for Real Medicine. Dr Thornton, both physician and herbalist, would face the challenge by lighting a cigarette and inviting his patient to drop his pants and bend over: 'Injections by the anus of the smoke or decoction of tobacco have been used with advantage in cases of obstinate constipation threatening ileus.'
And little risk of lung cancer, either.
See also **Putrefaction of the Excrement.**

Imposthumes or Abscesses
The mainstream treatment, as explained by Dr William Buchan MD, Physician to Her Majesty, in 1776[50], was quite straightforward: you made up a mercureal bolus, or large lump of a pill, based on that well-known poison, mercury: 'Make a diaphoretic mercureal bolus thus: take of calomel, six grains; conserve of roses, half a drachm; make a bolus thereof, and take over night with a glass of mercury in a watery mixture. For abscess, gangrene, cancer, ulcer and chancres [shallow ulcers], mercury is the only confirmed cure of these diseases.'
This prescription is not in the current issue of MIMS, which is just as well since conservation groups go environ *mental* if more than a millionth of a gram of mercury is found in a litre of drinking water – which means that the thirty or so grams of mercury that doctors then recommended as a night-cap could have polluted thirty million litres of drinking water, or one patient.
Although mercury is on the government's red list of twenty-three toxic subtances that are dangerous in the water supply, an environmentalist who went on television to frighten viewers about minute traces of mercury in some British drinking water appeared to have a mouthful of mercury-based fillings that did not worry him at

all. Medical anxiety has always been selective.

Imposthumes & Pernicious Mushrooms

The orthodox herbal remedy for humans was for centuries the garden mushroom (*agaricus Campestris*), as Nicholas Culpeper, the seventeenth-century herbal guru explained in his definitive work. Modern readers might be inclined to cavil in detail:

> This is much better than that which grows in the field, which is often unwholesome and pernicious. It owes its origin to the putrefaction of earth or dung.
> Mushrooms are under Mercury in Aries. Roasted and applied in a poultice, or boiled with white lily roots, and linseed, in milk, they ripen boils and abscesses better than any preparation that can be made. Inwardly, they are unwholesome, and unfit for the strongest constitutions.

Alternatives to mushrooms were oats and the garden onion. The porridge was to be mixed with vinegar and applied to 'hard imposthumes' in order to 'dissolve them'. The onions were beaten together with figs and applied as a warm poultice until the abscess ripened and broke; leaks did a similar job, they said, but took longer.

Inoculation, see Variolation

Itches & Breakings Out of the Body

Though not life-threatening, itches can be annoying – ask any television newsreader. The safe solution was of young hops, boiled and rubbed on to the part in question. Best bitter might work, but that is guess work.

J

Jaundice, Both Yellow & Black

Gardeners have always had trouble with alehoof, or ground ivy – trouble in eradicating it, that is. Yet earlier gardeners treasured it as a part of Real Medicine's armoury of plants, not alone in releasing that bile that otherwise seeps into the blood and makes yellow perils of us all: 'Boiled and drunk, it helps the yellow jaundice by opening the stoppings of the gall and liver.'

Garlic, eaten in lumps or spooned out as conserve, released the flow of bile and removed the jaundice, Culpeper said.

K

Kidneys

The formation of painful stones has long attracted the surgeon's skilled knife, but before that it attracted the equally skilled barber's razor, for they were '... stone cutters, bone setters, cataract couchers, herniotomists, pig gelders, midwives and surgeons.'

The duty doctor at one hospital rather patronizingly explained the current modality: 'these days we cut kidney stones with ultra-sound – a bit like Dire Straits played even louder,' she said. See also **Pissing By Drops**

King's Evil, The

The king's evil, or the king's disease, became royal and therefore socially acceptable after King Louis IX returned with it from the crusades in 1254. It reached England four or five years later. Usually it was no more than jaundice, but sometimes it was leprosy or scrofula.

Scrofula [*tubercular adenitis*] was painful, producing swellings and open sores on the face and neck; sometimes the sores became putrid, but it was rarely fatal, and, importantly from the marketing point of view, it was liable to natural remission.

Things started looking up when word got round that the royal touch would totally cure the disease. Since it did indeed tend to clear up if left alone, it only took the royal PR team to pick out a few such cases, extrapolate the statistics a little, and come up with a seemingly divine gift capable of founding a lasting myth.

The Plantagenets were great touchers, and accompanied their touch with alms, usually of one penny. Edward I was reported by his team to have touched 983 scrofulous subjects in one year, then to have increased his turnover to 1,219 in the following fiscal year, and to have peaked at 1,736 touched in the third year; in each case the touchee then touched the toucher for a penny.

The Stuarts had much better PR advice and took their publicity further, claiming that their gift was evidence of their family's divine right to rule absolutely everybody, while acting on their accountants' advice by holding on to their pennies. Queen Anne was the last royal toucher. Now she is dead, one hears.

Kupffer Cells

'Kupffer cells are the star-shaped cells present in the blood-sinuses of the liver. They form part of the reticulo-endothelial system and are to a large extent responsible for the breakdown of haemoglobin into the bile pigments.'[51]

This is the sort of fact that one is entitled to know.

L

Leeches for a 5 ml Suck

Wet cupping, surviving into the 1970s, roughly corresponded with leeching in that they both performed a similar task; they simultaneously frightened and reassured the patient, caused them manageable pain and did them no harm. Each leech was good for about five millilitres of blood exfusion. Breeding and supplying them was a sizeable industry. They surely will return to fashion before long.

Lethargy, & Garlic

If the humours of the body failed to circulate, the blood itself could become stagnant in the body, failing to ebb and flow as it was intended to; in some cases the brain could even cease making blood; or its electric charge could be vitiated by the fact that blocked perspiration sealed the body off from the *Orgone* or vital force of the universe on which it depended. True, one could then buy an Orgone Box, as one can today buy an ionizer, to allow the universal energies to enter the body, but the short cut was to eat garlic, for 'it helps the lethargy', Culpeper said.

Liver, Cooling When Heated
In ancient days the liver not only got itself jaundiced, it also tended to overheat; cooling it was simple, according to Culpeper: 'A syrup made of the juice [of young hops] and sugar, cures the yellow jaundice, and tempers the heat of the liver and stomach.'

When did you last feel your liver to check for hardness? Had you done so three hundred years ago, you would have been encouraged to know that 'A decoction of Horehound is available for those that have hard livers.'

In case you wondered, it softened the organ by 'opening both the liver and the spleen'.

Liver Growth, Curing
Doctors had no cure for this condition that they had not yet understood. Herbalists had: 'Pennyroyal [*Mentha pulegium; Hedeoma pulegioides* in the USA], being boiled and drank, purgeth the liver-growth.'

Lousy Evil, or Leprosy
Leprosy (Greek, scaly) was a term applied to many skin eruptions, including eczema, psoriasis, scabies and the burrowing of mites and lice. One common treatment for them all was to bruise mustard seed into honey, mix it with wax, and rub it on, for, 'it takes away the leprosy or lousy evil,' said Culpeper.

The Complete New Herbal, edited by Richard Mabey[52], echoes Culpeper's famous title and follows broadly similar lines, but without the blood-letting, opium, cannabis, witchcraft and astrology that made the barking mad old gentleman's original book so distinguishable from others. For psoriasis, the new herbal suggests: 'Herbal remedies which relax and strengthen the nervous system, such as skullcap, vervain, wild oats, passionflower, chamomile, and hops, can be included in a herbal prescription to treat psoriasis to good effect. Licorice may help to support the adrenal glands and a Bach Flower Remedy (Star of Bethlehem) can also be taken if appropriate.'

Dr Edward Bach's colleague, Norah Weeks, explained that he came upon his eponymous Flower Remedies when 'He became extra sensitive to his intuitive faculty, for he found that by holding his hand over a flowering plant he would experience in himself the properties of the plant.'

Lues

Commonly known today as syphilis, a symptom of which is a swelling in a lymphathic gland of the groin – known as a bubo. Mercury-based ointments and drinks were used to treat 'The Confirmed Lues with Buboes in the Groin', as well as the accompanying symptoms, such as 'Abscess; Gangrene; Cancer and Putrid Ulcers'.

'Mercury,' the medical books of the day attested, 'is the only confirmed cure of these diseases,' but it must be admitted that for almost any venereal disease mercury and some form of opium would be prescribed: ask Culpeper or any other respected herbal advocate. The usual method was to powder the seeds and add them to a drink, but the down side of this treatment was that it also had to be accompanied by bleeding under the correct star sign in order to draw the bad humours out of the body.

Lungs, Cold Rheums of the

There is no reason why a tall and scruffy weed should be any worse than a tall and scruffy doctor at curing chesty wheezes:

> The syrup of the Horehound [*Marubium Vulgare*] is excellent for cold rheums in the lungs of old people, and for those who are asthmatical or short-winded.
>
> Some praise the Black Horehound [*Balota Nigra*] very much as a pectorals in coughs and shortness of breath, but with this caution, viz, that it ought only to be administered to gross phlegmatic persons, and not thin plethoric persons.

How would an average GP's patients, now with access to their notes, react to being described as a 'gross phlegmatic person'? Or 'thin plethoric'?

M

Madness

Was madness a disease, and therefore an earner for doctors; or a possession, in which case it was an earner for vicars; or caused by a growth, needing the services of a lowly surgeon; or merely a chemical problem needing an apothecary's shrubs? Where did dissent from received perceptions end and madness begin?

The Anglo-Saxon Leech Book knew both the cause and the cure, neither, alas, without its detractors today; as in many Anglo-Saxon cures, the word 'drink' featured quite a lot:

> A drink for a fiend-sick man when a devil possesses the man or affects him from within with disease, to be drunk out of a church bell.
>
> Take githrife, yarrow, betony and several worts; work up the drink with clear ale, sing seven masses over the worts, add garlic and holy water, and drip the drink into every drink that he shall afterwards drink; and then let him drink it out of a church bell, and let the mass priest sing this over him after he has drunk it: 'Domine sancte pater omnipotens, &c.'

In an article on Sir William Paddy 1554-1634 in *Medical History*, there is the case in March 1604 of Mr Brian Bridger, a vicar, who, it was claimed, 'was a lunatic for claiming that Bishops that enforce men to subscribe to the ceremonies of the Church of England are therein anti-Christs'. Dr Paddy disagreed with this definition of lunacy, but it did not stop similar claims being made against John Wesley when he later set about the Church of England and its bishops with some enthusiasm.

Early psychiatry was also practised, to the amusement of doctors back in the seventeenth century. Dr Robert Fludd, 1574-1637, was a prominent Rosicrucian, who, his critics alleged, 'used a kind of sublime, unintelligible cant to his patients, which by inspiring them with a greater faith in his skill, might in some cases contribute to their cure. Bad demons caused diseases, and that the pious physician had to fight against them'.

Between demon-wrestlings he wrote *Medicina Catholica* in 1629, the first ever reference in medical literature in Britain to the circulation of the blood. Perhaps his haematology was better than his psychiatry.

Measles, or Mesel

Until Thomas Sydenham defined measles in 1670, the textbooks commonly used the word – 'mesel' in Chaucer – to describe leprosy, smallpox, measles, scarlet fever and diphtheria, and assumed that one common treatment would serve them all.

The commonest treatment was to immerse oneself in cold water to discharge the heat, and this still has its proponents today.

Medical Students, Seldom Useful Members of Society

Long hair, idleness, guitars, drugs, drunkenness, squalor, fornication, shiftlessness and a disrespectful attitude towards anatomical

samples – any sub-editor can write headlines about medical students.
A similar view was held in the eighteenth century, according to Dr
Buchan's later editions:

> 'A mere student is seldom a useful member of society.'
> 'Delirium, melancholy and every madness, are often the effect of close
> application to study.'
> 'All that man needs to know, in order to be happy, is easily obtained;
> and the rest, like the forbidden fruit, serves only to encrease his
> misery.'

One cure was to avoid listening to old whingers, like Bob Dylan
and Leonard Cohen, in favour of some upbeat stuff: '... to amuse himself after severe thought, by playing such airs as have a tendency to
raise the spirits, and inspire cheerfulness and good humour.'

Avenzoar of Seville [1072-1162] advised students that despite what
their textbooks told them it was nonsense to rely on astrology: 'The
wise scholars at Toledo contradict the assertions of astrologers, and
say that the art of medicine is based on observation and diagnosis.'

Melancholy

Melancholy was understood to result from an imbalance in the
humours, particularly, in this case, of the bile. Alehoof, or ground
ivy, treated melancholy, 'by opening the stoppings of the spleen'.
Shift the bile and there was no need for addictive tranquillizers.
Ground ivy flourishes wherever it senses that it is not wanted – like
grass and cats.

But it was Pennyroyal that got to the seat of the problem, for it
'purgeth melancholy by the stool,' although Nich. Culpeper also
wrote up garlic in psychedelic terms that seemed to suggest that it
combined the qualities of magic mushrooms, valium and Irish
whiskey:

> Authors quote many diseases that it is good for; but conceal its vices.
> Its heat is very vehement; and all vehement things send up but
> ill-favoured vapours to the brain. In choleric men it will add fuel to the
> fire; in men oppressed by melancholy, it will attenuate the humour,
> and send up strong fancies, and as many strange visions to the head;
> therefore let it be taken inwardly with great moderation; outwardly
> you may make more bold with it.

Menses, or Menstruation

The inner workings of women's bodies were always a source of
wonder to men in general and to physicians in particular. One thing
they knew was that each month a healthy young woman who was not
pregnant would menstruate, so any failure of the 'menses' or

'courses' to appear on time would call for a substantial plumbing job. Pipes had to be unblocked. Cisterns had to be flushed. Leaks had to be fixed.

Fortunately, there was one simple sample of Real Medicine that Dr Buchan claimed any man could make at home if he really wanted to get some faulty female plumbing working again: 'Take filings of iron, two ounces; cinnamon and mace, of each two drachms; Rhenish wine, two pints. Infuse for two or three weeks, frequently shaking the bottle; then pass the wine through a filter. Take half a glass two or three times a day. It would be as good if small quantities of vitriolic acid were added.'

If that seemed rather violent, there was a herbal remedy that simply involved eating garlic, for 'it provokes women's courses', but see **Melancholy** before eating garlic and driving.

See also **courses, Bringing down women's**

Mercury as Medicine
First note what Black was saying in 1971[53];

> The mercuric salts are all highly poisonous both to man and to bacterial life, so that they are strongly antiseptic. Taken internally, the first effect of the mercuric, and to a lesser extent the mercurous salts is by their irritating action to set up copious purging. They are also credited with the power of increasing the flow of bile, and for this reason the blue pill, which contains mercury, and mercurous chloride, i.e. calomel, were at one time much used as purgatives.

And what was the effect of administering this poison?

> MERCURY POISONING is of two kinds: (1) acute mercury poisoning, due to swallowing one of the soluble mercury salts, generally perchloride of mercury; (2) chronic mercury poisoning, produced either by continuing repeated medicinal doses of mercurials for too long, or by handling the metal or inhaling its fumes.
> *Symptoms* There is a burning pain, first in the mouth, then in the stomach, followed by diarrhoea and vomiting. The lips and mouth are generally burned white, and a metallic taste is left in the mouth. Great collapse soon comes on and the person may die in a few hours. If death does not take place at an early stage, the kidneys are liable to remain seriously damaged by the drug.
> When too much mercury is taken into the system in small doses, the first signs are an excessive discharge of saliva into the mouth, and tenderness about the teeth when the mouth is tightly shut. Next the odour of the breath becomes bad and the gums tender, spongy, and ready to bleed at the slightest touch, and the tongue swollen.
> Finally, the teeth become loose and drop out, the jaw-bone may

become diseased, the person becomes generally weak and bloodless, and may indeed die.

What treatment would they suggest?

'Treatment consists in stoppage of the mercury.'

So why the startage? It is difficult now to understand how mercury poisoning as medicine could have become as fashionable as it did, and how it could have outlived its victims; but, then, future generations may ask similar questions about amphetamines, tranquillizers and blood transfusions.

Mesmerism

Friedrich Anton Mesmer (1734-1815) was one of the world's top all-time quacks, combining audacious deception with astounding marketing skills. Not for him a pill or powder made from dried dog's dung or common chalk. His canvas was the universe, his power inter-galactic, his appeal, well, mesmeric. A contemporary account written in 1784 describes in delicious detail the astonishing trickery that made him a millionaire through his discovery of a marketable animal magnetism that trickled down from outer space through him alone:

> That there is a subtile fluid which fills the Universe; which constitutes a connecting medium between us and the heavenly bodies, and between us and earth. He said that this fluid is capable of receiving, propogating, and communicating impressions, at any distance, and that the consequent notions are subject to mechanical laws.
>
> He says he has discovered means by which he can direct the course of the fluid, accumulate it in one body and convey it to another at pleasure. And from its singular effects on Animal bodies, he has called it *Animal Magnetism*, as well as on Account of its having Poles like the magnet. He ascribes many diseases to the unequal distribution of it, and offers to cure many by restoring the equilibrium.
>
> His System, singular as it is, has more friends than enemies – his house is so much crowded that there are seldom fewer than two hundred people in it at a time, and that in succession from morning to night, all of whom undergo his operations. When you are told that he charges five guineas the first month, and four every subsequent one, from each patient; that he has already sold his Secret to above a hundred and fifty persons for a hundred guineas each, and that he cannot admit the number of Purchasers, they are so frequent, you will judge what an immense fortune he is likely to make in a short time.
>
> In the middle of his room is placed a vessel of about a foot and a half high, which is called here a *bacquet*, it is so large that twenty people can easily sit around it. Near the edge of the lid which covers it, there

are holes pierced corresponding to the number of persons who are to surround it. Into these holes, in the manner of Carra's experiment are introduced iron rods bent at right angles outwards, and of different heights so as to answer to the part of the body to which they are to be applied. Besides these rods, there is a rope which communicates between the *bacquet* and one of the Patients; and from him it is carried to another; and so on the whole round.

The most sensible effects are produced on the appearance of Mesmer, who is said to carry the fluid by certain motions of his hands or eyes without touching the person. I have talked with several who have witnessed these effects, who have seen convulsions occasioned and removed by a movement of the hand. In order to qualify this account, which will appear incredible if not ridiculous, I shall add the answer of Mr Le Roi the Academician to my question 'What he thought of it?' He has been appointed one of the Commissioners to examine into the operations of one *Deslon* who is a scholar of *Mesmer's*. His words were: 'Je n'en puis pas encore juger; mais j'ai déjâ vu des choses très singulières.' ('Too early to say yet, but I've already seen some very unusual things.')

Migraine, or Megrim

One looks first to *The Anglo-Saxon Leech Book*. One then quickly looks elsewhere hoping for a second opinion:

In case a man ache in the head, take the lower part of the crosswort, put it on a red fillet, let him bind the head therewith.

For the same: Delve up waybroad without iron, ere the rising of the sun, bind the roots about the head with crosswerts by a red fillet. He will soon be well.

For the same: Seek in the maw of young swallows for some little stones, and mind that they touch neither earth, nor water, nor other stones; look out three of them; sew up three of them in what thou wilt, and put them on the man that hath need: he will soon be well.

Once the headache had gone, there was no need to throw the magic stones away, for they had other uses: 'They are good for headache and eye-troubles, and for temptations of the fiend, and for night visitors [usually goblins], and for spring ague, and for nightmare, and for fascination, and for evil incantations. They must be big nestlings in which thou shalt find them.'

Later, opium was the principal pain killer for migraine sufferers, but there was more: 'For hemicranial headache with vomiting, try gentle purges, and a piece of flannel over the forehead at night, and take opiates.' Where did they get their opiates in those pre-codeine days? They made them at home with this simple Anodyne

Fomentation recipe: 'Take of white poppy heads, two ounces; elder flowers, half an ounce; water, three pints. Boil till one pint is evaporated, and strain off the liquor.'

Moon-Fall, the see **Quacks.**

Mountebanks
The mountebanks were first-division quacks, men with a shrewd insight into human psychology and the presentational skills of a pharmaceutical representative. The name comes from the Italian *monta in banco* from their need to jump up onto a stage in order to get the attention of the masses.

The most famous mountebank was Andrew Borde, a medical practitioner from Winchester, who counted Henry VIII among his patients. He was 'a celibatarian, drinking water three times a week, wearing a hair-shirt next to his skin and a sheet for burial at the foot of his bed.' He was also the original 'Merry Andrew', a sobriquet he earned from his prancing, jesting style of delivery at the fairs, markets and other places of public resort where he practised his craft of separating people from their groats. A nineteenth-century record describes the life of a mountebank in Tudor times[54] from earlier sources:

> Twice a day, that is, in the morning and the afternoon, you may see five or six several stages erected for them ... These mountebanks at one end of the stage place their trunk, which is replenished with a world of new-fangled trumperies. After the whole rabble of them has gotten up to the stage, the music begins, sometimes vocal, sometimes instrumental, sometimes both. While the music plays, the principal mountebank opens his trunk and sells abroad his wares. Then he maketh an oration to the audience of half an hour long, wherein he doth hyperbolically extol the virtue of his drugs and confections [medicines] – though many of them are very counterfeit and false. He then delivereth his commodities by little and little, the jester playing his part, and the musicians singing and playing upon their instruments.

Their style would seem familiar to anyone who had visited a modern-day street market or endured an alternative comedian's routine:

> The principal drugs they sell are oils, sovereign waters, amorous songs printed, apothecary drugs, and a commonweal of trifles. The head mountebank, every tiume he delivereth out anything, maketh an extemporeal speech, which he doth eftsoons intermingle with such savoury jests (but spiced now and then with singular scurrility), that

they minister passing mirth and laughter to the whole audience, which may perhaps consist of a thousand people.

In Ben Jonson's *Volpone* there is a description of such a mountebank at work in Venice and it is strangely reassuring to notice how little human nature has changed in all those centuries:

You all know, honourable gentlemen, I have never valued this ampulla, or vial, at less than eight crowns; but for this time I am content to be deprived of it for six: six crowns is the price, and less in courtesy I know you cannot offer me. Take it or leave it, however, both it and I are at your service! Well! I am in humour at this time to make a present of the small quantity my coffer contains: to the rich in courtesy, and, to the poor for God's sake.

Wherefore, now mark: I asked you six crowns, and six crowns at other times you have paid me. You shall not give me six crowns, nor five, nor four, nor three, nor two, nor one, nor half a ducat. Six pence it will cost you; expect no lower price, for I will not bate.

Another famous mountebank of the early eighteenth century might well have been the father of Victorian music hall's alliterative and hyperbolic performers. He traded as 'Watho Van Claturbank, a High German Doctor' although there were those who thought he might actually be a Dr Haines. A broadsheet published his peroration, which was a wonderful self parody:

Having studied Galen, Hypocrates, Albumayor, and Paracelsus, I am now the Aesculepius of the age; having been educated at twelve universities, and travelled through fifty-two kingdoms, and been counsellor to the counsellors of several monarchs. By the earnest prayers and entreaties of several lords, earls, dukes, and honourable personages, I have at last been prevailed upon to oblige the world with this notice, that all persons, young or old, blind or lame, deaf and dumb, curable or incurable, may know that they may repair for cure, in all cephalalgias, paralytic paroxysms, palpitations of the pericordium, empyemas, syncopes, & nasieties; arising either from a plethory, or a cachochymy, vertiginous vapours, hydrocephalous dysenteries, odontolgic or poragrical inflammations, and the entire legion of lethiferous distempers.

It affecteth the cure either hynotically, hydrotically, cathartically, poppismatically, pneumatically, or synedechnically; it mundifies the hypogastrium, extinguishes all supernatural fermentations & ebullitions, and in fine, it annihilates all nosotrophical morbific ideas of the whole corporeal campages.

Who could have refused the man his six pence after a performance like that? Even those who attended the markets realized that they were paying for his showmanship as much as for his potions, as can be seen in a diary entry of 1723 recording a sighting of a rich mountebank called Smith whose motto, rather wittily, was '*Argento Laborat Faber*' which does not mean 'My publisher has gone to work in South America' so much as 'Smith works for money':

He was dressed in black velvet, and had in his coach a woman that danced on the ropes. He cures all diseases, and sells his packets for sixpence a-piece. He erected stages in all the market towns for twenty miles around; and it is a prodigy how so wise a people as the English are gulled by such pickpockets. But his amusements on the stage are worth the sixpence, without the pills. In the morning he is dressed up in a fine brocade night-gown, for his chamber practice, when he gives advice, and gets large fees.

Another mountebank, Katerfelto, travelled throughout County Durham in 1790 'in a fine carriage, and attended by two negro servants in green livery, with red collars. In the towns he visited, these men were sent round to announce his lectures on electricity and the microscope, blowing trumpets, and distributing handbills.'

It was said that the crashing music drowned the cries of the patients, especially the ones experiencing enthusiastic piece-work dentistry without anaesthetic.

Murthambles, the, see **Quacks**

N

Nerves, The Truth at Last
Nerves, as every physician knew, were thin tubes containing a mysterious fluid which conveyed the orders of the soul to the body.[55] If it thinned, thickened or changed electrical polarity, problems resulted, so after emptying the patient, the thoughtful physician took care to incrassate, or thicken, this nervous fluid:

Besides these evacuants, repeated use should be made of anything that restores the nervous liquid and keeps it in its proper crasis; such as spirits of hartshorn, soot, blood, and sal Armoniac; in these cases I particularly recommend Balsam of Sulphur ...

Nothing affects the nerves so much as intense thought. It in a manner unhinges the whole human frame, and not only hurts the vital motions, but disorders the mind itself.

Or try digging the garden instead of watching late-night TV: 'We seldom hear the active or laborious complain of nervous diseases; these are reserved for the sons of ease and affluence.'

Or for women, according to Dr Buchan: 'Females are more liable to many diseases which do not afflict the other sex; besides, as the nervous system becomes more irritable in them than in men, their diseases need to be treated with greater caution. They are less able to bear large evacuations.'

New Disease, the

Young Edmund Verney was ill in 1657 and wrote to his parents, whose family gave us their delightful recollections as *The Memoirs of the Verney Family*: 'Truly I might compare my affliction's with Jobs'. I have taken purges and vomits, pills and potions, I have been blooded, and I doe not know what I have not had, I have had so many things.'

The poor lad was suffering from 'The New Disease', an epidemic that created a panic in 1657–8. Dr Denton, one of the age's most famous physicians, wrote to Edmund's father:

Blooding is the best thinge the surest and quickest he can yet doe, therefore I pray lett him have one yett. 3 full spoonfulls of the vomitage liquor in possitt drinke will doe well, and he may abide the same night when he goes to rest; let him take the weight of vi drachms of diascordium the next day, or the next but one; he may be blooded in the arm about 20 ounces.

The ladies of the time were less fond of huge blood exfusions, preferring a gentler treatment of an epidemic that they thought they could handle without any panicking male doctors. The Verneys' friend Lady Fanshawe wrote: 'It is a very ill kind of fever, of which many died, and it ran generally through families. While I suffered it I ate neither flesh, nor fish, nor bread, but sage possett drink, a pancake or eggs, or now and then a turnip or carrot.'

Another friend, Lady Hobart, also approved of non-blood management of the new disease, even her spelling did display an aristocratic disdain for correctness: 'If you have a new dises in your town pray have a care to yourself, and goo to non of them; but drink good ale for the gretis cordall that is: I live by the strength of your malt.'

Had there been a referendum on the matter, the beer would almost certainly have won against the 20-oz blood loss.

Oleum Magistrale

Every pharmaceutical manufacturer dreams of compounding a chemical product that will sell magnificently for generation after generation – like aspirin, Gee's Linctus, or Owbridge's Lung Tonic. As fast as they churn out the stuff, the cash keeps flowing in. A momentum develops, especially if some exotic ethnic quality could be attached to the product to enhance its mystic powers – like a diet sheet 'as developed for the Canadian Army', or anything 'formulated by the University of California', possibly for the all-conquering Swiss navy.

Just such a product was *Oleum Magistrale*. Although when George Baker wrote a book on the subject in 1574 he was merely re-opening an old can of Spanish worms, his narrative of distant Moriscos must have sounded tantalisingly foreign to his prospective British purchasers:

> The composition or making of the moste excellent and pretious oil called Oleum Magistrale. First published by the commaundement of the King of Spain, with the maner how to apply it perticulerly. The which oyl cureth these disseases folowing. That is to say, wounds, contusions, hargubush [arquebus?] shot, cankers, pain of the raines, apostumes, hemerhoids, olde vlcers, pain of the joints and gout, and indifferently all maner of disseases.

'All maner of disseases!' his readers exclaimed in rustic tones; 'that's exactly what I've got!' Baker thought it advisable not to give a full description of the distillation, for he was against divulging the new knowledge of chemistry to medical dabblers. He also left the names of the herbs in Latin, for he 'would not have every ignorant asse to be made a chirurgeon,' but he sketched in the Oil's impressive pedigree while taking a stisfying side-swipe at the dreadful Spanish:

> In the Realme of Spain there inhaybited a people called in the Spanish tung *Moriscos*, of the which nation there are a greater number in *Granado* and *Arogan* ... The Moriscos, although they be not as yet growen so suttle and crafty as the said Spaniards: yet neuertheless it hath beene well prooued and seen by experience that they haue had more knowledge then the said Spaniards, both in the secrets of nature, and also in the properties of herbs generally in the art of curing.[56]

So popular was it that the Spanish Parliament offered its inventor a pension of 30,000 maravedis for the secret of its manufacture. He replied in effect that he would rather continue selling golden eggs than part with the goose that laid them. So popular was it that local doctors took him to court as a quack and had him jailed. There was uproar from the people whose health and life, they were sure, depended on their having a regular supply of the oil, so they bailed him out.

The King offered him one thousand ducats for the formula, but he still declined to tell the secret to anyone, apart from his wife just before he died. She was then banned at the instigation of surgeons and others from making or prescribing the oleum, so she sold it on for a pension of 60 ducats, but as soon as the secret of its manufacture was out, it ceased to work as effectively as before, other than in the export market.

In the meantime, the Royal Hospital of Toledo said, in 1561, that it:

> ... cured big wounds in head and arms ... in five or six days' time ... in some cases it was not even necessary for them to stay more than two or three days in bed, and in some cases no time at all; some needed no draining nor additional drugs; patients were not maimed as happened with people treated by surgeons; the art of Aparicio's treatment was cheaper than what surgeons charged.

There were soon dozens of conflicting versions of the formula, all packed in the famous little lead pots. It no longer works.

Opium

Culpeper's ageless book *The Complete New Herbal*, as updated by Richard Mabey in 1988,[57] now lists the poppy seeds' qualities only from a twentieth-century point of view: 'Opium poppy: seeds' constituents: some 25 alkaloids (including morphine, codeine, paparerine, thebaine, narceine), meconic acid. Main uses: *Culinary*: in baking. The unripe seed capsules of the opium poppy are used for the extraction of codeine. It is the ripe seed of the poppy that we use in cooking.'

Culpeper the herbalist was a much more committed fan of opium, and urged people to grow it and to use it as a narcotic and analgesic:

> The Opium Poppy is *Papaver Somniferum*. It grows wild in Ireland, but it is cultivated in the gardens of England. It flowers during the summer. It is under the dominion of the Moon.
>
> The seed-vessels are the parts to use. Syrup of diacodium is a strong decoction of them, boiled to a consistency with sugar. The syrup is a gentle narcotic, easing pain, and causing sleep; half an ounce is a full dose for an upgrown man, for younger it must be diminished accordingly.
>
> Opium is nothing more than the milky juice of this plant, concreted into a solid form. It is procured by wounding the heads, when they are almost ripe, with a five-edged instrument, which makes as many parallel incisions from top to bottom; and the juice which flows from these wounds is the next day scraped off, and the other side wounded in like manner. When a quantity of this juice is collected, it is worked together with a little water, till it acquires the consistence and colour of pitch, when it is fit for use. Opium has a faint disagreeable smell, and a bitterish, hot, biting taste.

Dr Thornton, in his roughly contemporaneous work, gives this entry in his table of the proportions of opium in some compound medicines: 'Tincture of opium contains, in a drachm measure, about four grains and a half of purified opium.'

There were, he agreed, one or two side-effects at any dosage, as there are with most pharmaceutical products: 'An over-dose causes immoderate mirth or stupidity, redness of the face, swelling of the lips, relaxation of the joints, giddiness of the head, deep sleep, accompanied with turbulent dreams and convulsive starting, cold sweats, and frequently death.'

Bringing it in from Turkey, India or China was expensive, so the narco-barons of the Society for the Encouragement of Arts, Manufacturers, and Commerce sponsored a competition to grow it in Britain.

In 1814 they awarded their gold medal to Mr Jones of Fish Street Hill for producing 21 lb of solid opium from five acres of land in Enfield.[58] The adjudication said that the prize-winning opium was 'far superior in flavour' to the foreign stuff.

Childred harvested the crop with a tin cup 'having one handle, so contrived as to fix itself to a girdle fastened round his waist'. They used a 'common garden knife' to scrape off the opium and found that 'Dewy mornings are best calculated for this purpose.' Sunshine was bad for opium-gathering.

Although learned physicians recommended its use to 'increase the energy of the mind, the frequency of the pulse, and the heat of the body, excite thirst, diminish all secretions and excretions,' its users had an irritating tendency to die. This was where surgeons came in. Dr Thornton reported on one interesting post-mortem examination of a patient who had died despite very large and frequent doses of raw opium and had been opened up by a surgeon to find out why:

> In one case where I inspected the body [not, you note, 'my much lamented late patient, how can I ever forgive myself?'] after death, the inner membrane of the stomach was remarkably corrugated, and with some inflammation; but as large doses of sulphate of zinc and flour of mustard had also been taken [not, you note, 'been shoved down his throat by me, his doctor, how can I ever, etc.'], no inference can be drawn from these appearances.

Obviously the legal profession had not yet caught up with the medical profession, or all sorts of inferences could have been drawn.

This particular use of opium was standard practice at the time. Dr Thornton also recommended it[59] because it 'prevented inflammation, by relieving the spasms'. Should the herbalist – or magistrate – enquire, Culpeper's advice on cannabis is on page 40, on opium on page 88.

The social after-effects of this opium-pushing were illustrated in some of the Sherlock Holmes stories; for example, in 'The Man With The Twisted Lip' Dr Conan Doyle describes one of the opium dens which in the 1890s lined 'the north side of the river to the East of London Bridge':

> Between a slop-shop and a gin-shop, approached by a steep flight of steps leading down to a black gap like the mouth of a cave, I found the den of which I was in search. Ordering my cab to wait, I passed down the steps, worn hollow in the centre by the ceaseless tread of drunken feet; and by the light of a flickering oil-lamp above the door I found the latch and made my way into a long, low room, thick and heavy with the brown opium smoke, and terraced wooden berths, like the forecastle of an emigrant ship.
>
> Through the gloom one could dimly catch a glimpse of bodies lying in strange fantastic poses, bowed shoulders, bent knees, heads thrown back, and chins pointing upward, with here and there a dark, lack-lustre eye turned upon the newcomer. Out of the black shadows there glimmered little red circles of light, now bright, now faint, as the burning poison waxed or waned in the bowls of the metal pipes. The most lay silent, but some muttered to themselves, and others talked together in a strange, low, monotonous voice, their conversation coming in gushes, and then suddenly tailing off into silence, each mumbling his own thoughts and paying little heed to the words of his

neighbour. At the farther end was a small brazier of burning charcoal, beside which on a three-legged wooden stool there sat a tall, thin old man, with his jaw resting upon his two fists, and his elbows upon his knees, staring into the fire.

How could doctors have subjected their patients to such dreadful risks of addiction? Fashions change. As recently as 1960 the *British Medical Journal* (p.820) was able to speak lightly of giving potentially addictive uppers and downers to sick children: 'Amphetamine – or preferably dextramphetamine – is used as a routine by most neurologists to counteract any sleepiness due to phenobarbitone. Children (or adults) may find a dose of 2.5mg adequate.'

Is that the received view in the 1990s? Doctors act for the best, making the best use they can of new discoveries and new modalities. When experience proves them wrong, they change again. The practice of medicine will always be an imperfect art, not a precise science. Culpeper, Thornton and Buchan could not have foreseen the degradation and death that would have come from their confident and well-meaning use of what seemed to be a wonderful plant with curative powers.

Organ Transplants

According to a picture by Alonso de Sedano in the fifteenth century, two Arabic Christians, trading as Saints Cosmas and Damian, performed a miraculous leg transplant in the thirteenth century. Their leg job was a curious precursor of Dr Barnard's heart transplant in the 1950s in that in both cases the 'donor' was black and the recipient white. The anaesthetic then in current use by surgeons was either opium or mandragora, but were anaesthetics used for miraculous transplants? Adam was given one in the creation of Eve.

One of the more gruesome attempted organ transplants was early in this century when a German experimenter, E. Ullman, tried to graft a pig's kidney onto a woman's arm – or was it the other way round? In either event, his defence that she was suffering from uraemia at the time seemed pretty thin, especially when friends stopped inviting her round for dinner.

P

Palate of the Mouth, Fallen

What could you do if the palate of your mouth suddenly fell? Briefly, you could pour some black pepper on a drink of your choice, gargle with it, and zap! your palate sprang back into place with alacrity.[60] Also useful for mild hangovers.

Palsy

A palsy was, and is, a paralysis. The wasting palsy is now called motor-neurone disease, the dumb palsy may well have been a stroke, trembling palsy was probably Parkinson's disease, and lead palsy was induced either by working closely with lead – lead smelters, typesetters, plumbers, pottery workers, manufacturers of white lead, and so on – or, iatrogenically, as a result of taking too many medicaments that included this heavy metal in the prescription.

This was partly because in the early seventeenth century the general view of doctors had remained unchanged for a couple of thousand years: a palsy was all down to humours getting misplaced inside the body (metastasis). A letter from Dr John Symcotts to a patient in July 1633 explained the mechanics of it in patronizing-the-patients prose:

> The crick of your neck, the pain of your toe, the swelling of your knees and the trembling of your joints which you call the palsy are all from one and the same cause. The hotter temper of your liver is not only the fountain of the hot and sharp humour of choler surcharging the mass of blood, from whence comes the preternatural heat which you feel, but also that the serous watery humour (which dilutes the mass of blood and by his tenuity makes it apt to be carried from place to place) is unnaturally salt and sharp which, being an excremental part of the mass, is from the same separated and voided by urine, by sweat, or insensible transpiration.
>
> Now in case natural heat be languid and delayed (as in age it must

be) it is lodged in some sensible part, as among the nerves, muscles and membranes, and there by his unkindly qualities causes exceeding anguish and pain. From hence comes the sharp headache, the squincy [quinsy], pleurisy, backache, the sciatica, joint sickness and the gout, of which kind your disease is. The weakness of the stomach is from pain of other parts, which by sympathy affects the stomach.

It was all hogwash, of course, but being written in technical detail with total assurance made it sound convincing. But was there a treatment for this assumed metastatic dysfunction? Of course ...

The course which I have propounded to myself in your cure is this: first, by a gentle purgative to abate such serous and waterish humours which must necessarily abound in the first region by your sedentary life and so are the antecedent matter. Though great and sudden evacuations may well evacuate the offensive cause yet they can never alter that habit which the law of custom shall impose and it must be disannulled by ... degrees.

Patients have always been reassured by some finger-wagging about their lifestyle, and this doctor would have loved the jogging craze – all that shaking up and down of the humours would have kept the body's morbific matter in a state of constant stasis, unless interrupted by 'great and sudden evacuations'. Perhaps it did. Perhaps it does. Who knows?

Panaceas

They thought it might be sulphonamides, they thought it might be antibiotics, they now think it might be probiotics or genetic engineering, but Nicholas Culpeper knew of experiments by alchymists and philosophers involving celandines (*Chelidonium Major*) that just might produce a marketable wondrous cure-all, and perhaps he was right, if only anyone could understand what he was writing about:

I have read, and it seems to be somewhat probable, that the herb, being gathered as I showed before [according to astrological rules], and the elements drawn apart from it by the art of the alchymist, and after they are drawn apart rectified, the earthly quality still in rectifying them added to the *terra damnata* (as alchymists call it,) or *terra sacratissima* (as some philosophers call it,) the elements so rectified are sufficient for the cure of all diseases, the humours offending being known, and the contrary elements being given. It is an experiment worth the trying, and can do no harm.

Did he try the experiment himself, or was he holding out for commercial sponsorship? There appears to be no further reference in his work to this incomprehensible amalgam of astrology, alchemy, superstition and celandines, which was a pity, because if it worked it would have sold like hot flushes.

In 1633 Dr Stephen Brasnell published a small book rather snappily called: *Helps for Sudden Accidents Endangering Life. By which Those that live farre from Physitions or Chirurgions may happily preserve the Life of a True Friend or Neighbour, till such a Man may be had to perfect the Cure. Collected out of the best authors for the generall good.*

These are some of his cures for all known poisons:

'The Hoofe of an Oxe cut into parings and boyled with bruised mustard-seed in white wine and faire water;
'The Bloud of a malard drunke fresh and warme: or els dryed to a powder, and so drunke in a draught of white wine.
'The Bloud of a Stagge also in the same manner.
'The seeds of Rue and the leaves of Betony boyled together in white wine.
'Or take ij scruples (that is fortie grains) of Mithridate; of prepared Chrystall, one dram (that is, three score grains), fresh Butter one ounce. Mix all well together. Swallow it down by such quantities as you can swallow at once; and drink presently upon it a quarter of a pint of the decoction of French Barley, or so much of six shillings Beere. Of this I have had happy proofe.'

His top-of-the-bill, all-star panacea special, though, was unlikely to appeal to the modern-day patient, especially if that patient is a young girl in jodhpurs:

Take a sound horse, open his belly alive, take out all the entrayles quickly, and put the poysoned partie naked into it all save his head, while the body of the horse retains his naturall heat, and ther let him sweat well. This may be held a strange course, but the same reason that teacheth to divide live pullets and pigeons for plague-sores approveth this way of sweating as most apt to draw to itselfe all poysons from the heart and principall parts of the patient's body. But during this time of sweating he must defend his braine by wearing on his head a quilt.

Was this just any quilt, you were about to ask? Would a duvet have done as well? No, this 'Nightcap to preserve the Brain' was a medicinal quilt, possibly colour-matched to the dead horse: 'The quilt is to be made of a number of dried herbs, which are to be made into a grosse powder and quilt them up in sarsnet or calico, and let it be so big as to cover all the head like a cap, then binde it on fast with a kerchief.'

For families wondering what to do with the pony now that their daughter has discovered that boys are more interesting, this just could have been a green way of recycling the old hack.

A later age thought that breathing pure hydrogen would be a panacea, if they could only get the sulphur and other odds and ends out of it. When they did manage to purify the gas, illness still persisted, so they tried pure oxygen. Would this usher in the golden age of pure Health for All? A machine was developed in the 1790s that did seem to produce purish oxygen and then deliver it in more-or-less measurable doses to the paying patients; however, a tiny problem became apparent as the physician leaned over his patients to take a close look at the colour of the face (with hydrogen their faces had gone black eventually, with carbon dioxide they had gone a pretty blue, so what colour would oxygen produce?). Dr Thomas Genry, reeling back from the stench of burning facial hair, managed to write this admonitory note in 1794: 'The process for obtaining inflammable air should not be conducted by candlelight, otherwise the approach of the candle to the stream of air may occasion dangerous explosions. For the same reason, when a patient is inhaling inflammable air by candlelight, the candle should be kept as distant as possible.'[61]

We all know that oxygen is not, strictly speaking, an inflammable gas, but it was good of the doctor to stagger from the explosions to his writing desk to warn his surviving patients, for as a result, few if any operating theatres in Britain to this day administer oxygen by candlelight.

Panting of the Heart – see **Heart Disease**

Paraphrenitis
Dr Buchan in all his editions described this as 'inflammation of the diaphragm', because he was not happy with the trend to describe British illness in Latin and Greek. Informed consent, he said, was easier when the patient learned he was suffering from 'putrefaction of the excrement' or needed some 'Waterloo teeth' rather than being confounded by a string of classical polysyllabalisms. However, that said, he did not actually offer any treatment for paraphrenitis: it is possible that holding some cold dung against it might help. But which dung?

Peripneumony of the Lungs, or Consumption
The Tudor treatment was easily available to all at low cost, according to Dr Bulleyn's *Book of Simples*: 'Snayles broken from the shelles

and sodden in whyte wine with oyle and sugar are very holsome, because they be hoat and moist for the straightnes of the lungs and cold cough. Snayles stamped with camphery and leven, will draw forth prycks of the flesh.'

This prescription has since escaped from the doctor's surgery to make its home in French restaurants, where peripneumonies are, possibly as a result, quite unknown.

Herbalists and Real Medicine alike had little help for consumptives. Although it was not until 1890 that consumption came to be seen as a separate illness, there was plenty of advice from Dr Buchan a hundred years earlier on preventing it: 'As this disease is seldom cured, we shall endeavour the more particularly to point out its causes, in order that people may be enabled to avoid it.'

The principal causes of consumption, as we all know, were manifold:

> Confined air; grief; disappointment; anxiety; close application to the study of abstruse arts or sciences; great evacuations, as sweating, diarrhoea; giving suck too long [this comes as a puzzler on the page, given the way the letter S was printed then]; piles; sweating feet; a bone stuck in the throat; making a sudden change of apparel; frequent and excited debaucheries; late watching; drinking strong liquors; sleeping with the diseased; constantly leaning forwards or pressing on the chest like cutlers and taylors; breathing cold night air.

In other words it was a lifestyle disorder brought about by almost everything, so the key to prevention was removing almost everything from your lifestyle, for there was no cure as such, although a diet of oysters and asses' milk was believed to help allay the symptoms. And the razor and bucket? Of course, as Dr Buchan shrewdly pointed out in 1776:

> If the patient does not spit, he must be bled according as his strength will permit, and have a gentle purge administered.
> A mixture made of equal parts of lemon-juice, fine honey, and syrup of poppies, may likewise be used. Four ounces of each of these may be simmered together in a sauce-pan, over a gentle fire, and a tablespoonful of it taken at any time when the cough is troublesome.

This prescription might remind older pharmacists of the tendency some years ago for patients to become addicted to paregoric cough medicine and Gee's Linctus when they were also opium based. These unwelcome regular customers were gradually banned from pharmacy after pharmacy until they were driven to bribe other people to pop into Boots for a bottle or two. The effects of pure opium on our ancestors were socially devastating. See OPIUM.

Horehound (*Marubium Vulgare*) or Black Horehound (*Balota Nigra*) could be dried and boiled up with its seeds and a little honey to relieve the pain of coughing. But much curiouser was this tip, in a book written for medical self-help in British homes in 1769[62] by William Buchan: 'Take of spermaceti, a scruple; gum ammoniac, ten grains; salt of hartshorn, six grains; simple syrup, as much as will make a bolus. This bolus is given in colds and coughs of long standing, and beginning consumption of the lungs. It is generally proper to bleed the patient.'

Where did they get this waxy secretion from a sperm whale's head? There must have been a steady supply, for it featured in many prescriptions.

Periods, or Menses, & Iron Filings

There was a simple DIY remedy for any problems down under: 'Take filings of iron, two ounces; cinnamon and mace, of each two drachms; Rhenish wine, two pints. Infuse for three or four weeks, frequently shaking the bottle; then pass the wine through a filter and drink a half a glass two or three times a day. It would be as good if small quantities of vitriolic acid were added.'

It is mortifying to see how long it took doctors to realize that their treatment of some conditions actually made their patients worse. Whether it was heavy metal then or tranquillisers in the Sixties and Seventies, it has often been difficult for experience to outweigh the sheer mass of accumulated literature on popular treatments. Popular with practitioners, that is.

The seventeenth-century herbal approach to overflows was mellower: a few medlars (*Mespilus germanica*), picked when the fruit is bletted (over-ripe but not yet rotted, like the brains of mature students). They boiled the fruit in water and kept it bottled in case of an out-of-season attack. 'It is a good bath to sit over for women whose courses flow too abundantly, or for bleeding piles.'

This book could provide a distracting read while you crouch to have your healing sit.

Pestilence

This all-purpose word gradually vanished from medical terminology, but it was popular for a while, as in Dr Bulleyn's *Book of Simples*[63]: 'Figges be good agaynst melancholy, and the falling evil, to be eaten. Figges, nuts, and herb grase do make a sufficient medicine against poison or the pestilence. Figges make a good gargarism to cleanse the throat.'

Pharmacists, Including Apothecaries

Apothecaries were acutely aware that their title only meant

'warehousemen' and that their professional body was the Company of Grocers. To add injury to insult, they were also known as surgeons, or 'short coats', so their shop should logically have been found between the grocer's and the barber's.

The ancient Egyptian pharmacists wrote their own prescriptions. They stocked a lot of mercury, vitriol, absinthe, beer, verdigris, purgatives, enemas, cannabis and opium. They used bleeding, cupping, vomiting and dieting. Little changed until the eighteenth century, when some new items started appearing on the shelves[64]:

> Fowler's arsenic solution, Hoffman's anodyne, Gregory's powder, potassium chlorate, phosphoric acid, quassia [wood of the West Indian tree *Picroena excelsa* – bitter enough to make a pink gin], angostura bark [even better bitter], Canada balsam, logwood, and Thomas Dover's powder; some of these new remedies came from American Indian medicine.

The Incorporation of Surgeons only became a Royal College in 1778, and as late as 1833, only eight years before the founding of the Pharmaceutical Society, forty-three chemists, druggists and apothecaries in Edinburgh practised surgery and included the prefix 'surgeon' in their description. There was still a pharmacist who was also a surgeon and 'accoucheur' registered as late as the 1870s, though it is doubtful whether he was actually still plying the forceps.

In his article 'The Struggle to Reform the Royal College of Physicians, 1767–1771', Ivan Waddington traced the work of dedicated physicians who wanted to turn a trade into a profession and thereby raise the standards of patient care. He quoted a letter written to William Cullen, the president of the Royal College of Physicians in Edinburgh, from Adam Smith in 1771, outlining his wry views on the conditions of graduation at Aberdeen and St Andrews.

> The title of doctor is not so very imposing, and it very seldom happens that a man trusts his health to another merely because that other is a doctor. The person so trusted has almost always either some knowledge of some craft which would procure him nearly the same trust, though he was not decorated with any such title. In fact, the persons who apply for degrees in the irregular manner complained of, are, the greater part of them, surgeons or apothecaries, who are in the custom of advising and prescribing, that is, of practicing as physicians; but who, *being only surgeons or apothecaries*, are not seed as physicians. It is not so much to extend their practice as to increase their fees that they are desirous of being made doctors.

Van Swieten complained bitterly in the 1760s that patients were going to pharmacists for medical advice and were, in the absence of regulation, being killed off by these unskilled shopkeepers:

I had a young man under cure, who was not ignorant of the medical art. I gave him some doses of white precipitate and the first signs of an approaching salivation appeared. I was desirous, as usual, to desist from the further application of mercury, until I saw the progress of the salivation. The patient being dissatisfied and impatient with this delay, sent to an apothecary for five grains of Turbith-mineral unknown to me; and immediately swallowed that dose, with a design, as he said, either to cure or to kill himself ... I was, in three hours after, hastily called to succour the wretch, then at death's door.

In the twentieth century specializing has gone even further, but somewhere along the line surgeons have climbed higher while pharmacists are still presumably restricted to counting pills, selling glucose sweets and putting sticking plasters on cut fingers. The growth market was in pain killers like opium and hemp.

Phlebotomy, or Blood Exfusions

For centuries, monks had insisted on being visited by a barber once a month to have him slit open a vein and draw off fourteen ounces of blood into a bucket. Why? Menstruation-envy, perhaps? If so, did they also have to fake PMT?

Bleeding was so fashionable that even patients who had already experienced severe traumatic blood loss were bled again on admission to hospital. Dr Abernethy records one such case in 1808[65]:

On Thursday a lad of 17 years of age had his head pressed between a cart wheel and a post; by which accident the scalp on both sides was turned downwards, so as to expose the lower half of the parietal bones, and also part of the frontal and occipital bones. The peritoneum was in several parts stripped from the skull.

The scalp, being cleansed, was replaced, retained in its situation by strips of sticking-plaster, and a slight pressure by bandage was applied. The boy was perfectly sensible, his pulse regular, and not quickened.

He had bled considerably from the temporal artery, which had been divided by the accident; eight ounces of blood were, however, taken from his arm; and some purging medicine was administered each morning, which procured three or four stools. On Friday his pulse beat nearly 120 in a minute; his skin was hot and dry; and he complained of pain in the forehead.

Twelve ounces of blood were taken away, and four grains of pulvis antimonialis ordered to be given three times a day. On Saturday his symptoms still continued and were rather increased. The antimonial powder made him sick, or at least increased his disposition to be so. Fourteen ounces more of blood were taken from him; the vibratory feel of his pulse not being altered until that quantity was taken away.

On Sunday his pulse was lowered by evacuations using antimonial wine. The pain of the head remained as before. Having a sufficient number of stools [occupational therapy?] and the sickness still continuing, the antimonial powder was omitted. He was bled, however, in the vena saphena [the large vein that runs up the back of the leg to join the deep veins behind the knee: good flow of blood, easy to cut], and his feet and legs were afterwards immersed in warm water. A blister was also applied to his neck.

The result? Amazingly, this tough young man survived.

Phlebotomy – Fifty Times
How did the bloody practice of bleeding and leeching survive for so many centuries? One clue lies in the fascinating case notes of Dr Samuel F. Summers in 1770:

> With regard to repeated bleedings, it is certain that much benefit may be derived from the practice. Dr Dovar, who brought this practice into vogue about fifty years ago, did not hesitate to take away six ounces of blood every day for a fortnight, and then every second, third, or fourth day, until the patient had been blooded fifty or sixty times.
>
> In general, I have observed that the patients are sensible of more relief two or three days after the bleeding, than they are immediately after it.

Phlebotomy & the St Valentine's Massacre
Weird astrological rules gave the phlebotomy business a phoney credibility. Strangely, Al Capone must have known a thing or two about these rules, and it was just slightly possible that what might have been an act of medical solicitude on his part has been widely misinterpreted:

> If you submit to blood-letting on May 4 or 5, you will never be taken by a fever.
> In March and May blood should be taken from the right side of the body,
> In autumn from the left side.
> The feast day of St Valentine is especially propitious for blood-letting.

Perhaps it was Capone's 'massacre' that led to the decline of St Valentine's Day blood-lettings and the consequent rise of the card industry.

Phlegmatic Conditions
For no apparent reason, ordinary cheerful people could become cold, sluggishly indifferent to life's exciting challenges. Doctors explained that this was brought about by cold, moist phlegm, one of the body's four liquids or humours, produced by heat (Greek, *phlegma*, a flame;

phlegein, to burn). Herbalists went further and produced a cure: 'GARLIC is under Mars as well as the former. The root is only known in physic; it is a powerful opener, and on account of its subtle parts, in which it abounds, discussive. It seldom agrees with dry constitutions, but it performs almost miracles in phlegmatic habits of body.'

Phlogosis, with Intense Torture
The precise identity of this illness is no longer known, but it suggests a fiery, burning condition, possibly a cancer of the uterus. Dr Willis in the 1600s treated phlogosis with purges and blood exfusions, according to this letter to an enquiring colleague:

> The Curative intentions are very narrowly confined and comprise practically only these two aims, namely to sweeten the blood and meanwhile to draw off its wastes and dregs from the affected parts. Phlebotomy from the veins of the arms is to be used, and serves both intentions. And in a similar case I have known the following remedy to bring great help, namely that every month or six weeks, up to five or six ounces of blood should be let. In place of purging, the bowels should be loosened by the use of softening Enemas and now and then a gentle purge.
>
> If a draught of whey, with infused flowers of pale roses and correctives suit her, exhibit it every 7th or 8th day; or if through queasiness of the stomach Medicines are required in very small quantity I would prescribe pills of this sort, which contain nothing deleterious.
>
> Best Senna one ounce. Rhubarb 6 drachms, lemon sandal 1 drachm, salt of Absynth ½ drachm, yellow oranges 1 drachm; cut and pound. Infuse lukewarm in water of Fumaria for 13 hours. Strain. Evaporate to an extract in a very gently heated Bath, adding toward the end best Senna powdered 2 drachms, Rhubarb powder 1½ drachms, lemon sandal 1 drachm. Make a mass and form into pills. Dose 2 scruples to ½ drachm.
>
> Prepare this sort of distilled water, of which she is to take three to four ounces twice or thrice a day, sweetened with syrup, stuck on a pin and imbued with powder of white sugar.

If it was uterine cancer, the prescription was unlikely to be other than palliative, for Dr Willis then moved up a gear in his war on private pain:

> Leaves of hart's tongue, alchymilla, Pylosella, Plantago, Bugle, Tapsus Barbatus, of each three handfuls; rinds of 4 Oranges. On all this pour three pints of whey. Distill in a common vessel. It is perhaps fitting to lessen the pain that she should sit in a perforated seat and draw into the affected parts the fumes evaporating from the hot decoction of this kind:

Leaves of tapsus barbatus, 3 handfuls. Cook in spring water s.q. If pessaries can be used, smear them with an ointment of p populneum or linseed, or both mixed together and pounded till black in a large lead mortar.

But the best method of cure is to use milk or whey daily in large quantities, or (if obtainable) slightly acid waters, so long as they contain no pungency, like those drunk at Buxton in Derbyshire. Let her morning and evening drink ass's or cow's milk raw and mixed with the aforesaid distillation and sweetened with rose water or syrup of violets. At other times let her drink it cooked with bread or dehusked oats, adding a portion of spring water.

Piles, and the Trinity

John of Ardern [1307–90] became a specialist on haemorrhoids when he found a Real Medicine cure that has since been lost to medical science. Until now, that is: 'For the relief of Piles, write the name of the Trinity on a piece of paper with blood from the little finger, and say three Paternosters.' Only the most irreverent sufferer would wonder where the piece of paper was then to be put.

Folk medicine was pragmatic, if not dignified: 'Sit with your fundament in a cold river an half hour ... Bathe the Parts with cold tea.'

It is important to get this perfectly clear: sitting with your fundament *in* the river, or bathing your parts *with* cold tea effected the cure. Sitting *beside* a river while *drinking* cold tea was not so much a therapy as a picnic and probably anachronistic at that.

Another folk remedy of Wesley's day called for the greatest possible attention to detail in its preparation: 'Take some dried stinging nettles and compress them into the shape of a suppository. Insert it carefully, after making sure that the nettles are thoroughly and completely dried.'

Or, rather than risk embarrassment by having to explain to your family what it is that has just slithered down your leg to the floor, Culpeper's cure might have been safer: 'Take knapweed [*genus Centaurea*, a sort of spineless thistle], privet, or the tamarisk tree [a naturalized shrub growing on sea shores in southern England].'

In case you winced, it was not considered necessary to insert the entire tamarisk tree other than in really serious cases. Or, a painless alternative: 'Washing the fundament often with the juice of cinquefoil (*Potentilla*) will also relieve the itching, if you let it dry itself without wiping.' There is just one cavil – it did not work if Jupiter was feeling poorly at the time: 'If Jupiter were strong, and the moon applied to him, and his aspect good at the gathering, I never knew it miss the desired effect.'

Hound's tongue was also recommended for piles, but the less one knows about the ins and outs of that remedy, the better.

Cuckoo Pint, or Wake Robin (*Arum maculatum*), helped a bit: 'The leaves and roots boiled in wine with a little oil and applied to the piles, or the falling down of the fundament, easeth them, and so doth sitting over the hot fumes thereof.'

More conventional by far was this three-century old recipe for the relief of piles that could even be knocked up in the kitchen and sold to passers-by: 'Take of ointment, two grams; liquid laudanum, half an ounce. Mix these ingredients with the yolk of an egg, and work them well together.'

They need only have added a little garlic and some pastry, and they could have sold the left-overs to their young as narcotic pizzas. The ointment was to be applied morning and evening until the problem shrank. If, in the meantime, there was any discomfort, this home-made mega-codeine cocktail helped: 'Take of white poppy heads from the East, two grams; elder flowers, half an ounce; water, three pints. Boil until one pint is evaporated, and strain out the liquid. This will relieve acute pain.'

Pin and Web

This eye disease, mentioned by Culpeper, Shakespeare and others, seems to have referred to cataracts characterized by a small pin-like lesion and a weblike opacity (Greek, *cataracta*, a portcullis). Removal by knife or needle is an operation that goes back thousands of years, but John Gaddesden, who was royal physician at the court of Edward II early in the fourteenth century, left these instructions for others to follow. Such welcome insights into early surgical practice help us to understand why barbers' chairs always tipped back into the Sweeney Todd position:

> The patient should sit in front of the physician in a well-lighted place whilst the sun is shining and there is no shadow. His knees should be drawn up to his chest, and bound at the ends of his nose, opening the eye that is affected: meanwhile the assistant should hold his head, bent back slightly, and lift up the eye-lid.

So far this reads like a script for an Xmas panto, but, like a panto, it tails off badly:

> Then take the instrument or a steel needle with a sharp, round head, and begin to pierce from the side of the lachrymal gland in the conjunctiva, pressing it towards the two tunicles, penetrating the empty space of the eye which is in front of the pupil. And let the surgeon hold the eye until the perforation is complete, and press the needle down until it is hidden beneath the cornea.

There was more, but enough is enough. Even Dr Wesley's wacky wallow in alternative therapies seemed little worse than that horrendous experience: 'For films on the eyes take dried human dung, well powdered, and blow it into the affected eye.'

Culpeper believed that the celandine (*Chelidonium Majus*) was the answer to most eye questions, and ophthalmologists may be excited to rediscover this age-old non-surgical treatment for their private patients:

> The distilled water of celandine (*Chelidonium Majus*) with a little sugar and a little good treacle mixed therewith (the party upon the taking being laid down to sweat a little) hath the same effect; the juice dropped into the eyes cleanseth them from films and cloudiness that darken the sight, but it is best to allay the sharpness of the juice with a little breast-milk.

The evidence of the age suggests that relief was indeed experienced, so perhaps some bright spark should try synthesizing or marketing it. But why breast milk?

There was another common cure that had few side-effects: 'The water wherein the root [of Cuckoo Pint, or Wake Robin] hath been boiled, dropped into the eyes, cleanseth them from any film or skin cloud or mist, which begin to hinder the sight, and helpeth the watering and redness of them, or when by some chance they become black and blue.'

As a good herbalist, Culpeper was against surgical intervention on principle, and went on at some length about the advantages of celandines over scalpels, even in his barking mad astrological mode:

> This is an herb of the Sun, and under the celestial Lion, and is one of the best cures for the eyes, for all that know anything in astrology know that the eyes are subject to the luminaries; let it then be gathered when the Sun is in Leo, and the Moon is in Aries, applying to this time; let Leo arise, then may you make it into an oil or ointment, which you please, to anoint your sore eyes with: I can prove by my own experience and the experience of those to whom I have taught it, that most desperate sore eyes have been cured by this medicine; and then I pray, is not this far better than endangering eyes by the art of the needle?

Yes! Yes! the patients cried as they fled the hospital's waiting room for the horoscope-and-shrub shop across the road, anything is better than having needles poked into my eyes. Alas, as often as not they were driven back to the surgeon when the herbalist's celandine failed to do the trick: 'For if this doth not absolutely take away the film, it will so facilitate the work, that it may be done without danger.'

How much danger was there from physicians with their acids and
alkalis fizzing away in glass bottles? Culpeper feared them more than
he feared the surgeons:

> Another ill-favoured trick have physicians got to use the eye, and that
> is worse than the needle; which is to take away the films by corroding
> or gnawing medicines; this I absolutely protest against.
>
> 1. Because the tunicles of the eye are very thin, and therefore soon
> eaten asunder.
> 2. The callus or film that they would eat away is seldom of an equal
> thickens in every place, and then the tunicle may be eaten asunder in
> one place before the film may be consumed in another, and so be
> readier to extinguish the sight than to restore it.

For patients who had suffered iatrogenic blindness, he offered
some comfort from superstition mixed with subjective experience
drawn from experiments carried out on live animals:

> It is called chelidonium, from the Greek word *chelidon*, which signifies
> a swallow, because they say that if you put out the eyes of young
> swallows when they are in the nest, the older ones will recover them
> with this herb; this I am confident, for I have tried it, that if we mar the
> very apple of their eyes with a needle she will recover them; but
> whether with this herb or not I know not.

Pissing by Drops

Like piles, this painful condition elicits little sympathy. At least one
would know what the problem was with a good English name like
that, rather than having it called something foreign like enuresis.
Whatever they called it, 'piffing by dropf' could be cured the
Culpeper way by a day at the seaside: 'Sea holly is venereal, under
the celestial Balance. It cures French pox and piffing by drops.'

The cherry tree (*Prunus Cerasus*) also offered remedial aid: 'The
tart or sour cherries when they are dried, they are more binding to
the belly than when they are fresh, being cooling in hot diseases and
welcome to the stomach, and provoke urine.'

The French, of course, called French pox (*Morbus Gallicus*) the
English pox, but then they would, wouldn't they?

The Holy Thistle (*Carduus benedictus*) could be boiled into a
decoction that had a special cure for pissing by drops, since it reached
right into its astrological causation; it might be wise even now to ask
one's GP for more details should he prescribe holy thistle on
astrological grounds: 'It provokes urine, the stopping of which is
usually caused by Mars or the Moon.'

The 'red wild campion' had an impressive inter-planetary

reputation for easing the flow of urine and removing kidney stones:
'They belong unto Saturn; and it is found by experience that the
decoction of the herb, either in red or in white wine ... being drunk
helpeth to expel urine being stopped, and gravel or stone in the reins
or kidneys.' There were also two orthodox medical choices, including
mercury in handy home-made pill form: 'After the patient has first
been purged and griped, take half a drachm of mercurial pill night
and morning, or the mercury may be taken in liquid form, as it may
be suspended in a watery mixture.'

Should none of these be favourable to your horoscope, you could
call on the help of Mercury without using mercury: 'Wild carrots
belong to Mercury, and therefore break wind [why has Patrick Moore
never made this connection?] and remove stitches in the side, and
provoke urine.'

The seeds were better than the roots for medicinal use and they
caused less wind, Culpeper said. Or, turning to the professionals:

Take of calomel [Remember? Mercurous oxide, poisonous irritant
producing purging, flow of bile, diarrhoea, burnt mouth, general
collapse, death], and precipitated sulphur of antimony [a black irritant
powder, producing vomiting, purging, sweating, paralysis of the heart
and nervous system] each three drams; extract of liquorice, two
drachms. Rub the sulphur and the calomel well together; afterwards
add the extract, and mix with gum arabic and make into pills. Take two
or three, night and morning.

Dr Buchan's 'simple' was truly simple: 'The patient should walk
across a cold floor as often as possible, or he should take a
teaspoonful of sweet spirits of nitre.'

Sometimes the retention could be caused by trauma, and these are
susceptible to treatment by acupuncture, according to this anecdote
from Joshua Horn's *Away With All Pests* (Hamlyn, 1969):

The pelvic injury must have bruised the nerves to the bladder, for the
patient was unable to pass urine. To deal with this we called in a
colleague from the acupuncture department. The Chinese traditional
doctor, bearded and dignified, felt the pulse, nodded sagely, and in a
completely matter-of-fact way told the patient that his problem would
be solved immediately. This unbounded confidence in the efficacy of
their treatment is characteristic of traditional doctors, and probably
contributes not a little to their success.

He cleaned the skin with iodine and alcohol and, with a delicate
twirling motion, inserted five acupuncture needles into the chosen
spots. Within a few minutes the patient was able to pass urine and from
that time onward he had no further bladder trouble!

In 1982 Alexander MacDonald reported in his book 'Acupuncture' that traditional doctors outnumbered their modern colleagues by three to one in some Canton rural communes. In the 1960s they had been equally balanced, and back in 1949 95% of all Chinese doctors had practised the traditional arts, including acupuncture.

Plague
The origin of plague was a mystery to medieval people as they navigated the narrow swamps that served them as streets in their cramped and crowded cities. Even in the eighteenth century, with 'night soil' accumulating in the unpaved streets under a dusting of quicklime, with offal and filth thrown from waterless houses into the drainless streets, few inferences were drawn.

Thomas Sydenham, according to an article by K.G. Keele in *Medical History*, introduced a possible alternative to Paracelsus and his astrological theories of Aries the Ram and Pluto the Dog in his definitive book *Methodus curandi febres* in 1666.

> Maladies arise partly from the particles of the atmosphere, partly from the different fermentations and putrefactions of the humours. The first insinuate themselves among the juices of the body, disagree with them, mix themselves up with the blood, and finally taint the whole frame with the contagion of disease. The second are contained within the body longer than they ought to be.

In 1685, after two winters when the Thames froze solid, fevers occurred in plague proportions, and Dr Sydenham wrote: 'Changes in a constitution arose from certain secret and hidden alterations taking place within the bowels of the earth and pervading the atmosphere.' These 'morbific particles' were also identified by Robert Boyle in 1660: 'Mineral exhalations may not only affect human bodies by being drawn into the lungs with the air they swim in, but insinuate themselves into the pores of the skin ... I think it very possible that divers subterranean bodies that emit effluvia may have in them a kind of propagative or self-multiplying power.'

These subterranean bodies have not yet been identified. The hunt goes on. Meanwhile, Dr Thomas Willis (1621–75[66]) was more concerned with cure than cause when he wrote to his colleague Dr Hodges with advice on how to treat a wealthy lady who had caught the plague:

> I shall profer the use of some means that may be tryd without offence or much trouble to the patient, and possibly may afford her some good; in such a case as I apprehend hers to be I would advise that after her body is prepared by some evacuation either by vomitt or easy purgation. THAT every morning in bed she take four pills of the malat that is prescribd, and then have a fomentation applied to the stomach and hypochondria [under the short ribs] for half an hour or more, then

that she take about two ounces of the liquor prescribed, and lies in bed an hour thereafter, and sleep is shee can and be in a breathing sweat when shee rises to have her stomach and sides anointed with the ointment, and have a blew paper [mercury] smeared over with the same to lay all over the arms and compleatly.

But he make it of nine clysters [enemas] used frequently; if those things are too hott and cause a greater ebullition of humours in the stomach, I admit that she take the pills in bed and an houre after drink a large quantity of new whey, or possibly some mineral waters such as Tunbridge may be most proper for her. I shall next opportunity send you a powder I have whereby to prepare an artificial water in imitation of Tunbridge, and not unlike it in operation which works very largely to your self, and in best wishes to the good of your patient I remain, Sir, your most humble servt. Tho. Willis.'

Of the liquor that he prescribed for plague victims, Dr Willis said, 'It is mainly Peruvian bark, and a liquor containing lemon, gentian, carduus benedictus [a thistle] in white wine.' The ointment 'is lavender, tansies, orange rinds and fresh butter in Spanish wine'.

Applying the deodorant syndrome, public health officials of the eighteenth century concentrated on prevention when they suggested keeping plague away by masking the smell, and purging the body just in case any plague managed to infiltrate the flowers: this was Dr Buchan's strategy:

To keep the house free from infection, aromatic herbs are to be burned on the fire, and windows are to be closed in cold weather. Internal remedies to be taken, are, mostly powders from dittany [g. *Dictamnus*], pimpernel, tormentil [*Potentilla erecta*], roses and violets, drunk in a glass of wine, but also pills containing cicotrine aloes [a purgative], fumitory, myrrh, crocus and other ingredients, which destroy the poisonous vapours which have infiltrated the pores.

In all fevers with inflammation, as pleurisies, peripneumonies [seems to include influenza] &c, thin gruels, wheys, watery infusions of mucilaginous plants, roots, &c are not only proper for the patient's medicine, but they are likewise the best medicines that can be administered.

A herbal pharmacopoeia suggests among the products of mucilaginous plants such ingredients as Iceland moss, olive oil, linseed, almond oils, isinglass and powdered arrowroot; they act mainly as demulcents, soothing the alimentary canal.

Before the germ theory gained acceptance, some attempt at preventive hygiene was evident during the York plague: all infected garments were to be removed with a pair of tongs and thoroughly boiled; other items were fumigated in sulphur for twenty-four hours, but no one thought of drains.

The search was on for a preventative or a curative. Long before organ or tissue transplants [but see **Organ transplants**] made it possible to recycle accident victims, similar but messier ideas were already in circulation, like this fourteenth-century cure for plague:

> Take the brains of a young man that hath died a violent death, together with its membranes, arteries, veins, nerves and all the pith of the backbone; bruise these in a stone mortar until it becomes a kind of pap, then put in three fingers' breadth of spirits of wine, digest for six months in horses' dung, and take a drop or two in water in every day.

Given that people died on the second or third day in the case of septicaemic plague, or the fourth or fifth day with pneumonic plague, preparing this cure timeously over six months was more fraught than trying to find a chemist's shop open at night in a strange city. Another problem was that demand for violent young men's pith might well outstrip supply in time of pandemic plague.

Plague – Shut That Pore!
Talbott's *Medicine in Medieval England* summarized the then current methods in use for avoiding pandemic plagues.

> One's life must be sober, abstemious and in all things temperate. Hot baths should not be taken, lest, by opening the pores of the skin, the pestilential air should enter and infect the whole body. Fruit should not be eaten, and no food cooked in honey; wine should be drunk sparingly, but vinegar could be mixed with everything.
>   To keep the house free from infection, aromatic herbs are to be burned on the fire, and windows are to be closed in cold weather. Internal remedies to be taken, are, mostly powders from dittany [g. *Dictamnus*], pimpernel, tormentil [*Potentilla erecta*], roses and violets, drunk in a glass of wine, but also pills containing cicotrine aloes [a purgative], fumitory, myrrh, crocus and other ingredients, which destroy the poisonous vapours which have infiltrated the pores.

Pleurisy
Dr Buchan was all for the big bleed: 'A large quantity of blood let at once, in the beginning of a pleurisy, has a much better effect than repeated small bleedings. I suggest about twelve to fourteen ounces, with another eight to nine ounces taken twelve hours later. Even then there may be need for a third or even a fourth bleeding.'
   On the other hand, in the snappily entitled paper, 'The Metastatic theory of pathogenesis', in *Medical History* by Malcolm Nicolson (*Metastasis* – 'the transference of morbific matter from one part or organ to another') was this record from Gerard Van Swieten's

Commentaries on Boerhaave's aphorisms, proving that pleurisy was all the patient's fault even in the early 1700s[67]:

A man aged thirty-four was treated by his physician for the cure of a pleurisy; and with such success that the fever and the pain in his left side were so far reduced by the second day of the malady, that the patient thought himself almost completely cured, and neglected to observe any further cure or regimen, but with an event that at last proved fatal to him; for he lived afterwards in a languishing condition, and confessed he always perceived an abtuse pain in the part that was first affected.

Within a few weeks after his first illness he had a considerable swelling in his right leg, that again disappeared of itself; and another of the like sort shewed itself after that in the right side, and of a considerable magnitude, that again disappeared spontaneously. Lastly, a like tumour appeared in the right thigh, and while it there continued another swelling formed itself upon the inner side of the right arm, becoming soft and larger than one's fist. At length succeeded a dysentery, an ascites and anasarca, with weakness, and death closed the scene. [Proving?] This whole history informs us, that an inflammation of the spleen, being by the neglect of the patient not completely cured, degenerated into suppuration; and that the matter thence absorbed was by various translations, or metastases, deposited upon divers other parts, until at length, the whole mass of blood was corrupted with purulent cacochymia.

And serve him jolly well right.

Psychiatry, the Early Days

A paper by William F. Bynum on 'British Psychiatry 1780–1835', included Countess Harcourt's description of the treatment of George III when apparently suffering from delusions: 'The unhappy patient ... was no longer treated as a human being. His body was immediately encased in a machine which left it no liberty of motion. He was sometimes chained to a stake. He was frequently beaten and starved, and at best he was kept in subjection by menacing and violent language.'

He was also blistered, bled, given digitalis, tartar emetic, and various other drugs. Sanity continued elusively to evade him.

A consultant psychiatrist said that he only knew one joke about his profession, and he did not think that particularly funny although it made his patients laugh:

A consultant is someone who knows everything, but does nothing.
A surgeon is someone who does everything, but knows nothing.
A psychiatrist is someone who knows nothing and does nothing.

A pathologist is someone who knows everything and does everything, but too late.

Purging the Brain

Every part of the body could be vomited, opened, purged, sluiced or bulldozed until it was clean: but what about purging the brain? Poking moodily at his luncheon one day, Nich. Culpeper, Gent., had a slight mishap that distressed his wife and his table-cloth, but solved this otherwise intractable problem. 'Mustard seed is good ... to use it both inwardly and outwardly, to rub the nostrils, forehead, and temples, to warm and quicken the spirits; it purges the brain by sneezing, and draws down rheum and other viscous humours.' Dr Thornton, the fashionable MD, favoured snuff for the same purpose.

Putrafection of the Excrement

This is not a good thing to have. Its cure was jotted down by an ancient Egyptian doctor, or possibly embalmer, on one of the Ebers[68] papyri in about 1500 BC:

> If you examine a person who suffers in the region of the stomach and vomits frequently, and you find a protuberance in the anterior parts, and his eyes are tired and the nose is stopped, then say to him: 'It is putrefaction of the excrement, the excrements are not passing through the intestines'; prepare for him white bread, absinthe in large amounts, add to it garlic steeped in beer, give the patient to eat of the meat of a fat beef and beer to drink composed of various ingredients, in order to open both his eyes and his nose and to create an exit for his excrements.

Almost every item of that treatment – white bread, lots of absinthe, beer, fat beef – would cause modern doctors to peer anxiously over their bifocals at their putrefying patients, yet what will *their* patients look like in three and a half thousand years' time? See also ILEUS, knotted bowels.

Q

Quacks

We owe the word to the Dutch, whose 'kwaksalver' was one who boasted of his salves, or cures. Most quack remedies plugged on TV these days are mainly harmless, relying on the 15% success rate usually attributed to placebos. It was not always so, according to the plaintive tone of the introduction to Dr Buchan's bestselling 1794 edition:

> As matters stand at present, it is easier to cheat a man of his life than of a shilling, and almost impossible to detect or punish the offender.
>
> People shut their eyes, and take everything upon trust that is administered by any Pretender of Medicine without daring to ask him a reason for any part of his conduct. Implicit faith, everywhere else the object of ridicule, is still sacred here.
>
> We would wish to call the attention of mankind away from the pursuit of secret remedies, to such things as they are acquainted with.

Among the most successful quack remedies were 'Goddard's Drops' or 'English Drops' which appeared at the time to be panaceas – the equivalent in Charles II's day, perhaps, to the sulphonamides of the 1940s. They cured colds, smallpox, syphilis and other tricky bugs. So popular were they that the government planned to build a National Health Service on their use, if only they could persuade Mr Goddard to sell them the secret of manufacture. Mr Goddard was finally persuaded to do so for the then multi-million price of $15,000. He managed to emigrate with his loot before the government scientists discovered that the principal active ingredient was aromatic spirits of ammonia, or smelling salts.

Some quacks became known as 'greasers of pox' from their custom of treating syphilis sufferers by smearing them from head to foot with 'Saracenic ointment' allegedly brought back from the Crusades. It seemed very much like old hogs' lard.

Joanna Stevens invented a 'secret cure' for 'the stone' that had such near-miraculous results that in 1739 Parliament passed an Act which is unprecedented in medical gullibility: it undertook to buy her secret in the interests of the nation's health and well-being.

Only Joanna knew the secret ingredients of her wonder drug when she had offered to make it public for the sum of £5,000, an immense fortune. A vain attempt had been made to raise this sum by public subscription, but only £1,356 3s came in so an appeal was made to Parliament, a commission was appointed to look into the matter, and a certificate signed by the archbishop of Canterbury, sundry bishops, peers and physicians was presented to the House, declaring that they were 'convinced by experiment of the utility, efficacy, and dissolving power' of this true Real Medicine. The Act was passed. Joanna Stevens got her £5,000 and the nation got the secrets that it craved, in her own writing:

> My medicines are a Powder, a Decoction, and Pills.
>
> The Powder consists of egg-shells and snails, both calcined.
>
> The Decoction is made by boiling some herbs (together with a ball

which consists of soap, swine's-cresses burnt to a blackness, and
honey) in water.
The Pills consist of snails calcined, wild carrot seeds, burdock seeds,
asken keys, hips and hawes, all burnt to a blackness – soap and honey.

Archbishops, MPs and doctors reeled back in disbelief, the magic
evaporated like a baked snail, and from that day to this Joanna
Steven's powders have ceased to have any efficacy.

Orthodox doctors of the late eighteenth century liked to prescribe
Blackrie's Lixivium, because it 'dissolved the stone' according to Dr
Hemerdon. The Lixivium was compounded of potash and quicklime
dissolved in water, but it did the trick. Alas, like many quack
remedies, it, too, has lost its power to heal.

Some quacks sold mysterious cures whose recipe was secret; others
sold recipes that the punter had to make up at home. One recipe,
according to McGrew, was a panacea that excluded no illness
whatsoever from its range and was nasty enough to be popular: 'Mix
red coral with crabs' claws, calcined human bones, grease from a
hanged man's scalp; add live toads, powdered earth worms and goose
dung. This will drive away those evil spirits that induce illness.'

At least in those days there was a sufficiently long list of capital
offences to make sure that no shortage of hanged men's scalps ever
plagued the quacks.

An article on 'Material of Medical Interest in the Cromartie Papers
of 1612' in *Medical History* lists some more of the patent medicines
then on sale:

'*The Countess of Middleton's Plague Water*'
'*Snail Water*' – though it is unclear whether it was used to feed or to kill
snails, or whether it was made from them.
'*Dyot Drink pro Hymorrhoids*': 'Sasaporoll four ounces; red, whit and yellow
sanders [cinders] of each one ounce, carander, swet fennoll and Anna seeds,
of each one ounce.'
There were potions '*For Poysons by fumes of mercury for the Palsy*' – an
early recognition of the dangers of the mercury treatment that was to stay in
fashion for a further two centuries at least.
'*Gaskins Powder*' – made of powdered pearls, coral, ambergris and French
brandy-wine. It was good for every complaint, Mr Gaskin claimed, as he
chuckled on his way to the bank.

An enterprising entrepreneur trading in Maiden Lane, London, in
1685 made a claim that even today's Trading Standards people might
have trouble with: 'A one hundred percent cure for disorders as yet
unknown to the world – The Strong Fives, The Wambling Trot, The
Murthambles, The Moon's Fall, and the Hockogrockle.' This latter
may be the first recorded occurrence of the Devonians' word for

day-trippers who flood into the county from 'up the line'; a characteristic of grockles, whose diet is limited to fish and chips washed down with rough cider, is that they do indeed get the Wambling Trots. See also **Foreign Travel**.

Other privatized cures included 'The black extremities of crabs' feet, pearls, the venom of vipers, and a stag's heart ...' to 'strengthen the heart and all the noble parts' as a cure for smallpox, bubonic plague and the measles.

Some remedies that would cure 'Fevers Intermittent, Remittent, Inflammatory, Nervous' carried an impressive guarantee:

Read, Judge, and try,
And if you Die,
Never believe me More

which became perverted by sceptics to:

Before you take this Drop or Pill,
Take leave of Friends, and make your Will!

What, though, of Dr James Graham, who qualified in Edinburgh in 1770, and opened a 'Temple of Health and Hymen' in which bimbos danced and sang in flimsy costumes while 'aethereal balsams' were wafted over punters trying to combat a failure of libido? Was he a quack? Or merely too market-oriented?

In her work on the 1832 cholera epidemic in York[69], Margaret Barnet reported that public health officials had to resist an inrush of purveyors of quack remedies – including 'Vincent Greatrake, the Irish Stroker' – who had arrived to compete with the physicians who were treating the victims with 1.5 grams of opium about twice in twenty-four hours and one gram of calomel if the patients' bowels needed to be purged, with 'cautious' bleeding to relieve headache and muscle cramps. This had nothing to do with quackery, which is selling remedies knowing them to be useless.

Valentine Greatrake had made a fortune at home in Ireland with his 'magical' cures. He arrived in London, where he hired a large house in Lincoln's Inn Fields, whence 'great crowds of patients of all kinds and conditions crowded daily, all clamouring to be cured. He received them in their order with a grave and simple countenence.' He claimed, some time before he was executed for treason, that everyone:

... was possessed by a devil, and that by his prayers and laying on of hands the devil could be cast out. Lord Conway sent for him to cure an incurable disease from which his wife was suffering, and even some of the most learned and eminent people of the time were among his patrons. You can hardly imagine what a reputation he gained in a short time. Catholics and Protestants visited him from every part, all believing that power from heaven was in his hands.[70]

Other entrepreneurs rushed patent medicines to York in obedience to market forces, including Daffey's Elixir, Moxon's Effervescent Magnesium Aperient, Morison the Hygienist's Genuine Vegetable Universal Mixture – all advertised on the front pages of the York papers[71].

Morison's Pills were very well recommended, even after a mother gave six to her child who had cholera and still died. An inquiry decided that the deaths were not due to the pills: 'A more unfounded report was never issued,' wrote Mr J. Webb of the British College of Health. They were, he said, 'all-powerful but innocent'. They cured every known bowel complaint 'by easy upward and downward evacuations, as well as fenague, gravel, abscesses'.

Mrs Ann Swaine of Walmgate, York, was called in as an additional testimonial:

> The violent pains in my side could not be cured by The York Dispensary or by any medical man in this city, but fifteen Morison's Pills per night for three weeks caused me to quit such a quantity of bile and corruption from my stomach and bowels that I was a wonder to all who witnessed it [!]. I have now discharged my maid, do all my own housework and can walk ten miles a day.

The editor, after interviewing several doctors, cautioned readers that professional opinion recommended sending for medical aid immediately. Whilst waiting, the patient could safely take 'twenty drops of laudanum in a wineglass of brandy, but nothing else'.

A prominent German quack was Franz Mesmer, who died in 1815. He took up Culpeper's astrological view that human DNA was formed at the moment of birth under the influence of stars and planets and added to it the theory of 'animal magnetism', in which the punters stood round a large tub of chemicals, holding hands ['group therapy'] while touching an iron ring on the tubs. Magnetism flowed out to them and through them, making them feel better as they paid their bills.

He also hypnotized women, especially Parisiennes, and groped them enthusiastically, 'including the erogenous zones', until they felt better ['grope therapy']. He would not have prospered but for the fact that all the medical faculties bitterly denounced him, thereby ensuring his success. He fled France during the Revolution and practised in Switzerland, where the temptations were fewer.

James Graham's celestial bed in his Temple of Health (1780) deserves a book – even a series – to itself. The bed, built on glass pillars, was wired to move up and down while 'aethereal balsams' were wafted across impotent couples; music played, erotic scenes and pictures surrounded them, a sense of floating in space was imparted by the electric gadgetry. If that failed to make things perk up, Emma Lyon, later just a good friend of Horatio Nelson, came in to perform erotic dances until the impotent became potent and the childless conceived. He went broke, though, and turned to the manufacture of false teeth.

Franz Joseph Gall decided that just as physical action can build up a muscle – like cyclists' calves and chess players' index fingers and thumbs – so brain action caused bulges in parts of that organ. He thus became the father of phrenology.

An orthodox modern doctor who had pushed tranquillizers for years could sympathize with the puzzled populace: 'No two characters can be more different than that of the honest physician and the quack; yet they have generally been very much confounded. The line between them is not sufficiently apparent; at least it is too fine for the general eye.'

Quinsies

An outbreak of peritonsillar abscesses had herbalists rushing out to gather mushrooms, though not to eat: 'Their poultices are of service in quinsies and inflamed swellings. Inwardly, they are unwholesome, and unfit for the strongest constitutions.'

R

Rabies

Britain had a lot of dogs, and many of them were mad. Culpeper had dozens of herbal nostrums for dog bites, including Bitter-sweet, All-Heal (of course), Adders Tongue, Bistort, Mouse-Ear and Pennyroyal. The ancient Jewish Talmud took rabies very seriously.[72]

What is the remedy? Abaye said Let him take the skin of a male hyena (or leopard) and write upon it: I, so and so, the son of that and that woman, write upon the skin of a male hyena *kanti, kanti, kloros, G'd. G'd, Lord of Hosts, Amen, Amen, Selah*. Then let him strip off his clothes and bury them in a grave at the crossroads for 12 months of a year. Then he should take them out and burn them in an oven, and scatter the ashes.

During the 12 months, if he drinks water, he shall not drink it but out of a copper tube, lest he sees the demon and be endangered. Thus the mother of Abba ben Martha who is Abba be Minyumi, made for him a tube of gold [to drink out of].

The tube of gold or copper was preferred to a glass lest the sufferer saw a reflection of the dog that had bitten him, with the attendant risk of sympathetic re-infection. The Babylonian Talmud accordingly singled out mad dogs for special dispensatory treatment on the Sabbath: 'Rabbi Joshua ben Levi said: All animals that cause injury may be killed on the Sabbath. Rabbi Joseph objected. Five may be killed on the Sabbath, and these are they: the Egyptian fly, the hornet of Nineweh, the scorpion of Adiabene, the snake of Palestine, and a mad dog anywhere.'

See also **Toothache**

Ramsden Therapy
This almost mythological dietetic approach to health and happiness originated in the 1960s at White Cross in Guiseley, Yorkshire, whence it has drawn pilgrims from most countries of the world. It seeks to unite the ancient elements of sea, earth, air and fire in one symbolic meal, and through this combining aims to reunite its believers with the joy that comes from perfect union with our environment, or Gaia.

The sea is represented by fish, a central feature of Ramsdenism; river fish like trout or farmed salmon are not eaten by the true believers. The land is represented by the potato, which grows in the womb of the earth; by such pulses as peas, which flower upon its surface, and by the flour of ground wheat, in which the fish is mystically enwrapped as by the belly of the Life-Mother.

Fire is used to cook both earth-element and sea-element in separate but continuous cooking chambers, with either vegetable or animal oil used to pass the heat of fire to the food of sea and earth. The earth's mineral wealth is symbolized by the libation ceremony in which tiny crystals as the soul of the sea from the womb of Gaia (little more than sodium chloride) and dilute acetic is shaken over the food before it is eaten.

Early exponents of Ramsdenism believed that Air should be included in the Therapy, so they would eat the whole meal experience while walking along the road chanting, 'Harry Ramsden, Harry Harry, Harry Ramsden' between bulging mouthfuls. When the meal was wrapped in newsprint – trees experiencing the *paperness* of paper – few therapeutic diets could rival the pleasure and sense of inner wellbeing thus produced. The trip to Guiseley is well worthwhile.

Relaxation of the Solids

In 1808 Dr Buchan's *Domestic Medicine Modernized*[73] offered some suggestions on treating this arterial illness that even very old GPs are unlikely to be able to recall: 'A general relaxation of the solids from lack of exercise can be treated with steel filings, alum, dragon's blood, elixir of vitriol, or cold baths.' No cruelty to an endangered species was involved; dragon's blood is a red resin taken from a big tree found on the Canaries – *Dracaena draco*, of the Lileaceae, usually used for colouring varnishes. The only species endangered by Real Medicine was, of course, the human species.

Rheumatism

As its name suggests, for centuries rheumatism was believed to be a damp disease caused by watery deposits in the joints. The good news was that one cure stood supreme: 'From the observed qualities of wine, it must appear to be an excellent cordial medicine. Indeed, to say the truth, it is worth all the rest put together.' Cheers. There were external remedies, too, like rubbing yourself frequently with Spanish fly: 'Take of Spanish flies, reduced to a fine powder, two ounces; spirits of wine, one pint. Infuse for two or three days; then strain off the tincture.'

Dr Edward Barlow MD, physician of Bath Hospital, wrote a tract[74], plugging Bath waters for the treatment of gout, rheumatism and palsy; many still believe him, and the treatment 'works', but orthodox Dr Buchan preferred something a pharmacist could weigh out on his scales: 'Take of conserve of roses, two ounces; cinnabar of antimony, one and a half ounces; gum guaiacum, one ounce; syrup of ginger, a sufficient quantity to make an electuary. Take a teaspoonful two or three times a day.'

The key ingredient was antimony, valued by early doctors because it got things moving and let the patient know that he had been treated; this is how Black's 1951 edition described the effects: 'The preparations of antimony are all irritants; hence in large quantities they are poisons, producing vomiting, purging, and also paralysis of the heart and nervous system. In moderate amounts they stimulate secretions from the bronchial tubes, intestine, and skin, and thus ease a cough, move the bowels, and cause free perspiration.' All of which was enough to take the patients' minds off their rheumatic joints for two or three days.

Rheums in the Eyes, Hot

The principles were simple enough: if part of your body was hot, you cooled it; if it was cold, you warmed it; if it was dry, you damped it; if it was wet, you dried it. Hot sore eyes were traditionally treated with cucumber, either the still-popular slice on the eyes while relaxing on the chaise-longue, or Culpeper's more pharmaceutical preparation: 'When the season of the year is, take the cucumbers and bruise them well and distil the water from them. The face being washed with the juice ... is excellent good for hot rheums in the eyes.'

Rhinoplasty

What, doctors have always wondered, could be done for people who had lost their noses? There seemed to be three alternatives: (1) make an artificial one out of steel or wood: this was not cosmetically acceptable to most patients outside of Transylvania; (2) saw a nose off a 'donor' and glue it on to the punter's face (the right way up or they could drown when it rained): this 'allograft' approach led then, as it leads now, to rejection problems; (3) snip a bit off the patient's own body ('homograft') and glue it onto the noseless face: this could leave the patient with two bits missing instead of one. This was not in itself an insurmountable objection until that sad day when lawyers realized that hospitals offered more challenges than conveyancing.

A book entitled *An Account of Two Successful Operations for Restoring a Lost Nose, from the Integuments of the Forehead, in the Cases of Two Officers of His Majesty's Army, including Descriptions of the Indian and Italian Methods*, is now out of print and tantalisingly unobtainable.[75]

Further research led to an Italian cosmetic surgeon called Gasparo Tagliocozzi, who, in 1597, after failing to 'restore the appearance of patients who had lost their noses' by sewing on spare bits of flesh from other people, moved into homografts when he learned to stitch the patients' missing noses to their upper arms and strapping the patients into a harness that made movement impossible: little by little the upper arm and the un-nose grew together, when, with a snip, the two were separated and, abracadabra! the patient had a sore nose and a sore arm. But *a nose*.[76]

Rondelles

When a brain surgeon trephines a circle of bone from a patient's skull, he wonders what to do with it. Not so with the so-called Neolithic men, who not only performed successful brain surgery, as evidenced by trephined skulls with evidence of bone regrowth, but also had the nous to sell off the rondelles as lucky necklaces. The

National Health Service has bucketfuls of kidney stones at its disposal each year, and they would make tasteful lucky cufflinks, costume jewellery or worry beads. Or are we too proud to learn from these private-practice ape men?

S

Sciatica
This useful catch-all description of a nagging pain just *there* has made it possible to offer equally useful catch-all remedies, like this one of Culpeper's:

> The outward application upon the pained place of sciatica [of black pepper seed mixed up with sugar and honey to make a soft paste, or electuary], discusses [*sic*] the humours, and eases the pain; as also the gout and other joint-aches, or other parts of the body, upon applying thereof to raise blisters, and cures the disease by drawing it to the outward parts of the body.

'Drawing it out' has always been a popular phrase with populist experts.

Scabies
In his 1547 book *Breviary of helthe* Andrew Boord wrote of scabies: 'In latin it is named Scabies. In English it is named scabbes which is an infectious sickenes, for one man may infect another by lying together in a bedde, and there be two kindes, the drye scabbes and the wet scabbes, or moist scabbes.'

Scurf
Dandruff still provides an unrivalled sales opportunity for drugs companies and quacks alike, and the beauty of it is that however much muck the sufferers buy and wipe on, as often as not they still have the problem, so still come back for repeat prescriptions. The *Complete Herbal* showed how to handle dandruff in the privacy of your own hedge, but with no shrub-back guarantee: 'The fresh roots [of Wake Robin, *Arum maculatum*] bruised and distilled with a little

milk, yieldeth a most sovereign water to cleanse the skin from scurf, freckles, spots, or blemishes, whatsoever herein. Authors have left large commendations of this herb you see, but for my part, I have neither spoken with Dr Reason nor Dr Experience about it.'

The modern view is that this itch is caused by a minute parasite, the *Sarcoptes scabiei*, which is attracted to our fingers, buttocks, genitals and feet, and confirms the danger of sharing a bed with itchy people. The solution then was a scrub in the bath, cleanish underclothes and a change of sleeping habits.

Scurvy in Sailors
The usual mortality rate on the convict boats to Australia was about 25%. The main cause was scurvy, brought about by a deficiency of vitamin C, or ascorbic acid, in the food. Contemporary captains' logs also pointed to lack of ventilation, exercise and sanitation for the prisoners, as well as reliance on salted food.

The bad conditions produced fetid breath and dysentery, which in turn fed the scurvy, or scorbutus. John White, who as surgeon-general to the fleet in 1790 accompanied one such ship on its doleful journey, insisted on adequate sanitation, fresh air, regular exercise and fresh vegetables for convicts and crew alike. He finished the trip with only 5% mortality, and had fruit and vegetable gardens planted in the settlement camp before he returned home. He had proved that scurvy was one of the easiest diseases to treat or to prevent. He also discovered that astringent resins from the Australian grass-tree (*Xanthorroea spp.*) and the red mahogany tree (*E. resinifera*) were effective healers, even taking a supply back to Britain with him for use there. He also found out that colic could be treated with oil distilled from the leaves of Australian eucalyptus trees (*Eucalyptus globulus*); it was, he said, far more efficacious than the English *Oleum Menthae Piperitae*. Generations of bronchitis sufferers gratefully inhaled its fumes. With Sir Donald Bradman, eucalyptus oil is probably Australia's most splendid contribution to modern life.

Secretions of the Chylopoietic Organs
In 1825 the clipboard on the end of the bed had not yet been invented, so doctors tended to forget what the patient in bed three was there for; he might pause for chat, ask after the patient's nose and entirely forget that he was an emergency accident case in need of intensive care. This was not desperately important, since the relevant facts usually emerged at the post-mortem examination:

> A gentleman fell with his leg between the bars of an iron grill, which served as a window to a cellar. The part was much bruised, the skin

grazed, and the tibia broken into three or four pieces at its upper extremity. The limb was put up in a splint by a neighbouring surgeon, and the next day the patient requested to see me in consultation.

I attended for a few days, but everything went on so well, that I discontinued my regular visits, and only called occasionally, without seeing the limb[!]

The patient seemed to be recovering well, sitting up in bed, playing cards and being ignored. Four weeks went by with no further examination of the leg:

The patient suddenly became delirious, and I was sent for to meet the other surgeon in consultation. The delirium was then so great, that the patient knew not the persons in the room.

On looking at the leg, with a view to enquiring into the cause of this unexpected occurrence, it was found, that one of the ulcers of the skin, on which his position had produced some pressure, had become deep, and apparently penetrated the fascia, so as to communicate with the fractured bone, and this had converted a simple into a compound fracture. To this event, we could not but attribute the sudden irritation of the constitution, and the delirium.

Opium was immediately given, which quieted this disturbance in a considerable degree, so that on the next day the pulse was more tranquil, and there was no delirium. On the following day, his stomach was affected; he was sick and had the hiccough, and his abdomen was distended. In this state he continued about twenty-four hours, when his sufferings were terminated by death.

In this case the disease was of too short duration [four and a half weeks] for observations to be made respecting the secretions of the chylopoietic organs [possibly the lymph glands, possibly not – just one more illness to worry about]; but it was evident that there was a complete atony of the stomach and intestines.

Shaking of the Mother

In medieval times doctors knew what to do with a tricky or extended labour: two of them lifted the mother off her feet and shook her up and down until something landed on the floor. This sometimes had perturbing results.

Skin, Diseases of

Leprosy was a principal skin disease, partly because any incidence of scaly skin (Greek – *lepros*, scaly) was called leprosy. The last native leper in Britain died in the Shetlands in 1798.

When Mr Martin Kelly, aged 40, reported to the out-patients' department of the Middlesex Hospital in 1761, Dr John Brisbane MD[77] carefully listed his symptoms before coming up with a firm diagnosis. You try, and see how you get on against the professionals:

his skin had dry scales 'from the crown of his head to the sole of his foot', the scales were 'thin and of all sizes', he 'collected two hatfuls from his body every day', he had no fever or other symptoms, and the scales were at their worst in the winter. Imagine what the wretched man's wardrobe looked like by the end of the week if his 'leprosy' was as bad as that – if it was leprosy. Just as unrecognizable gastro-intestinal upsets can be readily called 'a virus', so leprosy could serve in those days of Real Medicine as an alternative diagnosis to 'give in'.

Treatment? Correct again if you guessed three pints of camomile tea each day, three warm baths a week, two doses of Glauber's Salts a week, and a few teaspoons of antimonial wine each day. The leprosy cleared up, Dr Brisbane reported with a surfeit of hubris, but, inexplicably, it tended to recur in spring and autumn. Scalded skin was treated with a simple ointment made of olive oil, wax and sugar of lead, mixed together and cooled. The lead salt formed a whitish glaze on the burn, protecting it from infection.

Smallpox

There was no warning, no known cause, no practical prevention, no cure, so, said Boccaccio, the rich fled and the poor died. Miles Coverdale translated his sermon on plague in 1537 under the title: 'How and whether a Christian man ought to flye the horrible plage of the pestilence.' The answers, not to spoil it for the reader, were 'rapidly' and 'yes'. The next stage, borrowed imperfectly from Moses' words on quarantine, were included in these Tudor rules of 1574:

> The right Worshipful Sir John Sauage, Knight, Maior of the City of Chester had consideracion of the present state of the said cite, somewhat visited with what is called the plage, and divisinge the best meanes and orderlie waies he can ... within the cite aforesaid (through the goodness of God) to avoid the same, hath with such advice, sett forth ordained and appointed the points, articles, clauses, and orders folowing:
>
> That no person nor persons who are or shall be visited with the said sickness, shall go abrode out of their houses without license of the aldermen of the ward such persons inhabite, And that every person soe licensed to beare openlie in their hands ... upon paine that eny person doynge the contrary to be forthwith expulsed out of the said citie.
>
> The watchman to apprehend and take up all night walkers and such suspect as shall be founde within the citie.

Even the size of the licence was defined, and where on the body it was to be displayed; expelling miscreants made sure that the pox would still rage, but Not In My Back Yard.

What confused the attempts to prevent smallpox was the belief that it was caused by smells and that overpowering them would provide a cure. By the eighteenth century, much of the Tudor rigour had been replaced by a pragmatic desire to wash one set of bed clothes rather than a dozen, as Dr Buchan observed: 'Laying several children who have the small pox in the same bed has many dire consequences. The perspiration, the heat, the smell, all augment the fevers. They should be given a good wine, which may be made into a negus, with equal quantities of water.' It is easy to forget how widespread this infectious disease became, and how tough some of the treatments were. Dr Buchan in 1794:

This disease, which originally came from Arabia, is now so general, that very few escape it at one time of life or another. It is a major contagious malady; and has for many years proved the scourge of Europe. I have known children, to appease the anxiety of their parents, bled, blistered, and purged, during the fever.

Through ignorance of the causes and absence of effective prevention or cure, the pox raged unchecked, with frequent announcements in the newspapers like this one of 1744:

WHEREAS the Town of BURY ST EDMUNDS, where the GENERAL QUARTER SESSIONS of the PEACE of that Division are usually held, is now afflicted with the Small-Pox, for which reason it might be of exceeding ill consequence to the Country in General to hold the Sessions there; This is, therefore, to acquaint the PUBLIC that the next GENERAL QUARTER SESSIONS of the Peace will be held at the sign of the PICKEREL in IXWORTH, on Monday next.
Cocksedge, Clerk of the Peace.

Some newspapers carried weekly reports on the number of cases in each town, so great was the effect on life and trade.

Nov. 4, 1755.
Upon the strictest Inquiry made of the present state of the SMALL-POX in BECCLES, it appears to be in eleven houses, and no more, and that the truth may be constantly known, the same will be weekly advertised alternately in the Ipswich and Norwich papers by us,
Tho. Page, Rector.
Osm. Clarke, and Is. Blowers, Churchwardens.

See also **Variolation & Inoculation**

Snuffing, & Its Effects on Appetite for Dinner
Beleaguered tobacco companies, ever seeking new outlets for their deadly product, should take up Dr Thornton, the botanist and

herbalist, who, in an 1810[78] text book, reported on the role of snuff among early weight watchers:

> I knew a lady who had been for more than twenty years accustomed to take snuff, and that at every time of day; but she came at length to observe, that snuffing a good deal before dinner took away her appetite; and she came at length to find, that a single pinch, taken any time before dinner, took away almost entirely her appetite for that meal. When, however, she abstained entirely from snuff before dinner, her appetite continued as usual; and after dinner, for the rest of the day, she took snuff pretty freely without any inconvenience.

Soreness of the Breasts
In the dark days before pharmaceutical conglomerates, most prescriptions could be made up in the average kitchen: 'Sore breasts should be treated with a warm poultice of bread and milk[79].'

Spiders & Pill Bugs
Primitive or cottage medicine, typified by John Wesley's methodical collection of West Country cures, mixed superstition with magic to produce some very nasty ideas that nevertheless 'worked':

Take three large spiders and swallow them whole, one at a time, each day until the ague ceases.

Cut a large slice from a raw onion and bind it about the stomach for three days and nights, renewing the onion as necessary.

Roll cobwebs up into the size and shape of a doctor's pill. When you have six of them, make the child swallow them together for a certain cure.

From a damp and dark place under a stone or rotted tree take several pill bugs ('Isopod crustaceans of the genus Oniscadae' if this is a private consultation; 'wood lice' if it is on the National Health). Be reassured by the wisdom of the ancient saying, 'Spare the isopod and spoil the child', and swallow them when they are rolled up. This is rarely known to fail.

Spina Bifida & Spina Ventosa
These conditions were both clinically described by Rhazes, the Persian doctor who taught at Baghdad University and later at Cordoba: he died in 925 without having got further than a description. This impresses doctors, who much prefer his *Liber medicinalis ad Almansorem* to anything that Agatha Christie ever wrote, perhaps because he said: 'Truth in medicine is an unattainable goal, and the healing art described in books is much inferior to the experience of thoughtful physicians ... He who interrogates many physicians will commit many errors.'

Spitting Blood, & Marmalade

Gargling with marmalade seemed to cure this carpet-ruining condition: 'Soak seville orange peel in several waters, till it loses its bitterness; then boil in a solution of double-refined sugar in water, till it becomes tender and transparent. Then gargle with it.'

Sternutatories & Sudorifics

Real Medicine was brilliant at emptying the body. They used every orifice in order to drive out bad humours, evil demons or, later, such nasties as refined sugar or white flour. William Heberden the Elder was a prominent physician of his age, and he aptly summarized his working methods: in his *Commentaries* by William Heberden from 1802 onwards, recently written up by Ernest Heberden: 'One of the first considerations in the cure of a disease is, whether it require any evacuations; that is, whether it have been the general opinion of practical authors, that emetics, cathartics, diuretics, bleeding (by leeches, cupping-glasses, or the lancet), sudorifics, blisters, issues, sternutatories, or salivation, have in similar cases been found beneficial.'

A sudoriphic was something to drive humours out through the pores in the form of sweat, or – for private patients only – perspiration. A sternutatory had a kind of religious background in its ability to rid one's body of unwelcome extra-terrestrial possession by sneezing: demons could have had few nastier experiences than being expelled at eighty miles an hour from someone's nose in a mess of mucous. A cathartic was, and is, yet another term for a purgative.

In the Tudor era Dr Cassius wrote a taunting tirade against amateur practitioners who used these techniques while claiming mysterious exotic provenances. Patients, he said, should be at least as careful in their selection of doctors as they were of their cobblers:

Seek out a good Phisicien, and knowen to haue skills, and at the leaste be so goode to your bodies, as you are to your hosen or shoes, for the wel-making and mending wherof, I doubt not but you wil diligently search out who is knowne to be the best hosier or shoemaker in the place you dwelle: and flee the unlearned as a pestilence, to the comune wealth.

As simple women, carpenters, pewterers, brasiers, sope ball sellers, pulters, hostellers, painters, apotecaries (otherwise than for their drogges), avaunters themselves to come from Pole, Constantiple, Italie, Almaine, Spaine, Fraunce, Grece, and Turkie, Inde, Egipt or Jury: from ye service of Emperoures, kinges, and quienes, promising helpe of al diseases, yea, uncurable, with one or two drinckes, by waters six monethes in continualle distillinge, by *Aurum potabile*, by drynckes of great and hygh prices ... like to them which thinke farre foules have faire fethers, although thei be never so evil favoured and foule.

Stinking Breath

There was a lot of bad breath about in the seventeenth and eighteenth century, much of it iatrogenic. Physicians used mercury for more and more conditions despite its poisoning effects.

Death was a side-effect. All medicines have a side-effect or two, it is called a cost-benefit equation.

The herbal cure, also used by physicians of the era, was to drown the smell of stinking breath with something stronger – the ongoing deodorant syndrome. Top substitutes for halitosis in the days of Real Medicine were wild mint, rosemary and smallage.

For difficulty in breathing see **Asthma.**

Stomachs, Strengthening in Old People

Mr Culpeper had useful suggestions for older customers who could not take too much roughage, and for younger customers whose ambition was to be old one day: 'The roots of the carraways eaten as men eat parsnips, strengthen the stomach of old people exceedingly, and they need no to make a whole meal of them neither, and are fit to be planted in every garden.'

For customers who tired of caraway-parsnips, he had a sweeter prescription: 'Carraway confects, once only being dipped in sugar, and a spoonful of them eaten in the morning fasting, and as many after each meal, is a most admirable remedy for those that are troubled with wind.'

Stomachs, Weak

The most debilitated rake could toughen himself up stomach-wise with a little mustard:

> Black Mustard [*Sinapsis Nigra*] grows freely in waste places, and among rubbish; and is frequently sown in gardens. It flowers in June.
>
> Let such as have weak stomachs take of mustard-seed and Cinnamon, one drachm each, beaten into powder, with half a drachm of powdered mastic and gum-arabic dissolved in rose water, made into troches [lozenges] of half a dram each in weight, one of these troches to be taken an hour or two before meals. Old people may take much of this medicine with advantage.

Strong Fives, the, see Quacks

Suffocation of the Matrix

An interesting observation by a thirteenth-century gynaecologist had a distinctly male viewpoint: 'The types of women most likely to suffer from Suffocation of the Matrix [womb] are Virgins and Widows, whose natural instincts have had no outlet.'

This long-lasting male belief that all women's problems came from a lack of nooky and could therefore only be remedied by lots and lots of nooky has not been taken up to any notable extent by female physicians and surgeons of our time. Not that they have much opportunity of reaching the higher echelons of the profession; they are still, professionally, mere women, as is shown by the fact that only ten per cent of top medical appointments in 1991 went to the 'weaker' sex.

Surgeons

Avenzoar of Seville [1072–1162], according to the *Encyclopedia of Medical History*, liked to point out that whereas medieval physicians went home neat and tidy in their best pin-striped smocks, surgeons staggered home drenched in blood, exhausted from sawing, chopping and rebating. What was the answer, if you wanted to be a surgeon but did not want to get polluted with gushings and oozings? Delegation, of course. His career advice was simple:

> All operations, such as phlebotomy, cautery, incision of arteries, etc., should be assigned to assistants. And to them should be left even more important operations such as incision of eyebrows, lifting veins which enlarge the white of the eyes, and cataracts. The noble physician should do nothing but give advice about the medicine and diet of the patient, without undertaking any kind of manual operation, just as it is unseemly that he should make syrups and electuaries with his own hands.

What else was the humble pharmacist for, pray? In any case, it might have been naively optimistic to assume that all surgeons then could tell an artery from a vein. Quite a few of the more determined patients did survive, however.

William de Congenis, a privatized surgeon of the thirteenth century, wrote his advice from bitterly learned experience, to save other surgeons who might otherwise attempt, for instance, surgery on wounds of the liver:

> I advise the surgeon not to tamper with them: but you should tell the patient's friends that it may be fatal. But if the friends do not wish the patient to die without something having been attempted by the surgeon, demand a high fee, so that if you suffer the shame of seeing your operation unsuccessful, at least you will not suffer any financial loss.

The profession really came into its own with the European rediscovery of the ancient Chinese invention of gunpowder. Any half-trained barber could have cut out an arrow head or stitched up a spear wound, but gunshot wounds called for sterner stuff and more skilled intervention. The first book for surgeons dealing with artillery wounds came out in 1497 and tried to move its readers away from cauterizing wounds and amputations with hot irons, boiling pitch, or boiling oil of elder. Enthusiasts, who had borrowed the book, soon set up business behind the lines in M*A*S*H-type tents, offering cash operations – satisfaction guaranteed or your amputated limbs glued back on.

About this time Abroise Paré showed that vascular ligation of arteries could stop blood loss without killing the patient. This meant that for the first time surgeons could have regular customers. He also showed how to perform a herniotomy without chopping everything else off as well, thereby making future generations possible.

How did surgeons gain their skills? By practising on cadavers. Most barber-surgeons were totally reliable with a corpse, but first they had to find one. The *Encyclopedia of Medical History* has this eyewitness account of John Knyveton, a London medical student in 1752, doing some part time work to pay his fees:

> The graveyard was a large one, but we had marked the site of the grave and so found our way to it with tolerable ease, one of the young men however catching his knee against a Tomb Stone and severally damaging his Patella, or Knee Pan, at which he did swear lustily. Then to dig, and by our numbers soon uncover the coffin; and so to burst it open and drag out the body within, this being a man of some forty years, very well developed, at which we were well placed.
>
> Then to drag off his shroud, and the moon comes out faint from behind a cloud and shines on us, at which one Young Gentleman drops his spade with a great clatter and cries out with a Fearful Oath that it was his cousin, who had, it seems, been a Highwayman but lately caught and hanged. So we stuff the Body in the Sack, he muttering away beneath his breath; and so with some Relief of Spirits out into the Lane again.'

Understandably, in 1511 an Act of Parliament was passed to establish minimum professional standards by keeping out the illiterate, ignorant and female:

> WHEREAS the science and cunning of Physic and Surgery is exercised by a great multitude of ignorant persons, of whom the greater part have no manner of insight in the same, nor in any other kind of learning – some also can read no letters in the book – so far forth that common articifers, as smiths, weavers and women, boldly and accostumably took upon them great cures, and things of great difficulty, in which they partly used sorceries and witchcraft, and partly

supplied such medicines unto the diseased which are very noisome, and nothing meet therefore; to the high displeasure of God, &c.

Surgeons and Side Wards

Being shunted into a side ward and left for a few weeks while the waiting list gets prioritized is not a new problem. Dr Abernethy's patients knew all about this procedure[80]:

A man had the scalp bruised and torn down from off the frontal bone by the wheel of a cart. He was not stunned by the accident. The bruised scalp mortified and the bone was left bare. He remained in the hospital waiting for exfoliation and as he had no illness, but little attention was paid to him.

After about two months, however, he became weak and died; on examination an abscess containing one and half ounces of pus [Have you ever, in all your life, weighed pus? What would a handful weigh? Approx?] was found in the frontal lobe of the cerebrum, beneath the dead bone, and a full half inch from the surface.

Surgery, Brain, Tips on Performing

Dr Abernethy's notes give an interesting insight into surgical procedures in the eighteenth century. When an accident patient presented with a fractured skull the initial examination sounds fairly orthodox, but after that it changes:

A lad of eighteen was admitted with his temporal bone beaten in; the fracture ran horizontally, about a quarter inch above the zygoma. The upper part of the bone was depressed about an eighth of an inch, and it was impossible to trephine below the fracture in order to elevate the depressed portion. The lad recovered from the immediate stunning occurred by the injury; nor was there any symptom.

Surgeons and Theatre Sisters

The theatre sister then had to lay up a trolley for the great man: what did the trolley look like? Something like this: one bucket, metal, one razor, wiped cleaned on skirt, one bottle laxative, to wit rhubarb, aloes, senna, castor oil, one blister pad covered with mustard, one rag and one back-up rag. The surgeon then set about his patient:

He was bled largely, and took a purging medicine. On the second morning, he was again purged; and when I saw him at noon nothing appeared materially wrong; but when I came to the hospital at 8 in the following evening I found he had gradually become delirious, and that he could hardly be kept in bed. His pulse was frequent and strong. [? Action]

He was therefore immediately and largely bled. He now became quiet and manageable; but the next morning his replies to all questions

were incoherent [but we can guess what he was trying to say]. The
bleeding and purging were repeated, and at night a blister was applied
to his neck. [Of course]
   On the following morning he was fleeping and feeble. [? Leave well
alone] As his pulse increased in the evening, he was again bled.

The bucket was then emptied and possibly rinsed, whereupon it
was determined that brain surgery was no longer indicated. Dr
Abernethy in his 1825 notebooks also posed an interesting
intellectual conundrum for his fellow surgeons to ponder: 'An
operation performed on a healthy patient is more apt to produce
considerable disorder, than when performed on one whose
constitution has previously sustained the irritation of a disease, for
which the operation became necessary.'

Swimming, or Bathing

Broadly speaking, anything that was fun has always been opposed by
medical doctors. Dr Samuel F. Simmons went so far as to produce a
tract in 1770 warning people of the folly of sea bathing, back in the
days when the sea was made up of water, specifying such associated
perils as 'bursting a blood vessel' and 'inflammation of the brain'; he
also gave this peevish warning to recidivist swimmers:

> Yet, what is very remarkable, these people resort in crowds every
> season, to the seaside, and plunge in the water without the least
> consideration. No doubt they often escape with impunity, but does this
> give a sanction to the practice?
>   Unless the body has been previously prepared by bleeding, purging,
> and a spare diet, this can only be disastrous. If there is pain of the
> breast or bowels, or prostration of strength, or violent headaches, the
> sea bathing ought to be discontinued.

Imagine a beach with some of those pre-swimming services on
offer.

Swinging, Therapeutic

If you accepted the proposition – as everyone did – that most medical
disorders could be sorted out with a good session of vomiting, then an
intriguing question came up as well: was there an alternative to
chemical or herbal emetics? Those with no marketing skills would
have suggested a rough sea trip on a short and wallowy boat, but
where was the repeat business? And why share your profits with
scurvy sailors?
   Dr Thomas Beddoes, according to a piece by Dorothy A.

Stansfield[81], found just what the market was looking for, and in April 1794 he wrote an enthusiastic letter to Dr Darwin with the exciting news: yes, there was a way of inducing nausea that was quite different from boring old emetics. You could whizz them round on a machine until they were sick, and then charge them for it: 'If swinging could be perform'd by being placed on a chair, and whirl'd circularly and horizontally, so as to induce sea-sickness once or twice a day, even without vomiting by it, it might like real sea-sickness promote absorption – which is the means of curing self-spreading ulcers.'

He then got rather personal about his experiences when swinging with Mrs Kerr:

> When Mrs Kerr and I felt a glow at the head and the feet, the revolutions were near or above 100 per minute. At this rate we never felt any vertigo, but when the motion was slower, we did, the eyes being shut. When Mrs Kerr thought she slept better, the motion I know was slow, but I know not how slow – the nurse turning in the night – certainly not above 25 in a minute – She has still been free from flushing, except one evening, for a month past – You ask what alterations we have made – they were alterations for local adaptation. But there is an alteration which I thought wd. be an improvement, viz, to make the side pieces perpendr for the sake of more swinging – The pulleys are still as by your drawing. I should think if the heart were in the centre of motion, it wd be advantageous – It might in some cases, if the head were.

The machinery, which was made in Birmingham, underwent several modifications, but the underlying assumption remained true, that the body's humours could run off from where they were meant to be – as it might be, the pancreas – and end up somewhere where they should not be – as it might be, the lungs. So if you whizzed the patients around a fair bit, the likelihood was that they would get all the humours back where they belonged. It is difficult at this distance to follow this logic, as one would expect the victims to end up with all their humours packed into their head and feet. However, we are not doctors, let alone swinging specialists. Mrs Kerr, alas, slowly died, but she died excited and happy on Dr Beddoes' roller-coaster: 'The evening heats & flushes did certainly go away for weeks after this plan was entered upon and still keep away – and no known change in diet or medicine beside. Mrs Kerr is extremely weak – & gets weaker, but has no distressing feelings. Even her cough does not hurt – no chills, no sweats, hardly any flushing. It is the slowest decay I have seen.'

This was no mere aberration, for even J. Carmichael Smyth FRS, Physician to the King could write thus in his book *An Account of swinging* in 1787:

To conclude: as the sedative power of motion, to which I have ascribed the efficacy of sailing and swinging, is a principle hitherto unknown, I have been at some pains to establish it; and am convinced in my own mind [they always were], that when conducted with skill and integrity, it will not only be found useful in the cure of pulmonary complaints, but may probably be employed with advantage in a variety of other cases, especially when what is suggested shall have been improved by the ingenuity and experience of future ages.[82]

Alas, we have let him down. Now only astronauts know this thrill.

T

Technology

Anyone familiar with the technology in an intensive care unit would feel at home on Concorde's flight deck. Flickering digital readouts, oscillating dials, beeping electronics and masses of sellotaped wires worry the relatives and reassure the medical staff. 'The green numbers have gone from thirty nine point five to forty two point one,' says a worried father, unsure whether the figures relates to blood pressure, temperature, respiration or the price of burgers in the surgeons' snack bar. 'She's going to be all right, you can go home now, there's no reason to hang around here tonight' says the doctor yet again, stepping over them to flick a switch on an oddly after-thoughtish unit stuck on top of an untidy heap of apparently disparate machines, and nodding sagely as it beeps twice. The parents stay determinedly on, their eyes flicking from dial to dial, trying to read good news into their unblinking message as earlier parents had tried to read the entrails of a sacrificed sheep. Twas ever so, as Dr Buchan presciently bemoaned: 'The instruments of medicine will always be multiplied, in proportion to men's ignorance of the nature and cause of diseases; when these are sufficiently understood, the method of cure will be simple and obvious.'

Will men ever know the nature and cause of disease? Whenever one asks scientists the question 'Why?', they answer the question 'How?' Early doctors with their theories of astrological causation, morbidity particles and acts of God, were very suspicious of early microscopes that seemed to show worms swimming about in everything from blood to water. K. Dewhurst's work on Dr Thomas Sydenham, (Wellcome History of Medicine Library, 1966) recorded his views on microscopes in the 1600s: 'Nature performs her operations on the body by parts so minute and insensible that I think noebody will ever hope or pretend even by the assistance of glasses or any other invention to come to a sight of them and to tell us what organicall texture or what kinde of ferment ... separate any part of the juices of the viscera.' He added, on discoveries by Power and Hooke that these wiggly wormy things were discrete micro-organisms: 'They contribute very little towards the discovery of the cause and cure of disease.'

Clearly, intense scientific research by intense scientific researchers was not the answer, regardless of the question. Laboratories should be replaced with special licensed bars, according to Dr Buchan's views of his youngers and worsers:

> Nothing affects the nerves so much as intense thought. It in a manner unhinges the whole human frame, and not only hurts the vital motions, but disorders the mind itself.
>
> [Prescriptions] containing about fifty ingredients are still to be found in some of the most reputable dispensatories. As most of their intentions, however, may be more certainly, and as effectually answered by a few glasses of wine or grains of opium, we shall pass over this class of medicines very lightly.

Teeth & Dental Hygiene
The herbal route to dental hygiene in the days of Real Medicine involved the humble celandine: 'The juice or decoction of the herb gargled between the teeth that ache, easeth the pain, and the powder of the dried root laid upon any aching, hollow or loose tooth, will cause it to fall out.'

Teeth, Loss of
In the absence of dentists, and with little interest from physicians, the country cure for foul gums or decaying teeth of pressing strawberries against the gums held sway. Dried strawberries would do as well, so Nich. Culpeper included dried strawberries in his garden Pharmacopoeia.

Teething
Dr Brisbane's observations included these musing notes: 'I allude to the effects of the irritability of teething upon the health of children. The brain is sometimes so affected as to cause convulsions; the digestive organs are almost constantly disordered.'

Tenesmus
Sufferers from tenesmus experience symptoms similar to dysentery,

tumours and piles all at the same time; it is now viewed as a symptom of disease in the intestine, but centuries ago it was an embarrassment that called for help from the Cotton Weed, Cudweed, Chaffweed or Dwarf Cotton – *Gnaphalium Vulgare*:

> Venus is lady of it. The plants are all astringent, binding, or drying, and therefore profitable for all defluctions ... and to stay all fluxes of blood wheresoever, the decoction being made into red wine and drunk, or the powder taken therein. It also helpeth the bloody flux, and easeth the torments thereby; and being drunk or injected for a disease called tenesmus, which is an often provocation to stool without doing anything.

The broken-hearted sufferers were glad to know that Pliny, that famous mumpologist, had also insisted that Cudweed was 'a sovereign remedy against mumps'.

Testicles, Hardness of
Without providing us with a hardness index to use as an indicator, Culpeper offers a means of softening them up if that seems to be in order: 'The seed of Mustard of the Hedge (*Sisymbrium Officinale*) is good for ... hardness and swelling of the testicles, or of women's breasts.' They mixed it with honey and sugar into a syrup and drank it or just rubbed it on, simple as that. Or, if you grow beans in the garden:

> If a bean be parted in two, the skin being taken away, and laid on the place, it easeth both pain and *swelling of the testicles*.

Tetters
Like many forms of eczema, it was easier to allay the symptoms than investigate and remove the cause. One common cottage treatment was a decoction of young hop sprouts, picked as soon as they appeared in March, and rubbed onto the skin. Alternatively, for those seeking to effect a cure: 'The young hop sprouts, which appear in March and April being mild, if boiled and served up like asparagus, are a very wholesome as well as a pleasant spring food. They purify the blood, and keep the body gently open.' This is not dissimilar to present-day treatment, unless the patient happens to be allergic to hops, in which case Horehound could be tried: 'The green leaves bruised, and boiled in hogs'-grease into an Ointment, heals the bites of dogs, abates the swollen part and pains that come by pricking thorns; with vinegar, it cleanses and heals tetters.'
  For the Astrologico-Herbal treatment for tetters and most skin maladies Nich. Culpeper turned to a very special plant:

It is called Carduus Benedictus, or Blessed Thistle, or Holy Thistle. I suppose the name was put upon it by some that had little holiness in themselves. It is a herb of Mars, and under the sign of Aries. Now, in handling this herb, I shall give you a rational pattern of all the rest; and if you please to view them throughout the book, you shall to your content find it true ... It strengthens the attractive faculty in man and clarifies the blood, because the one is ruled by Mars. The continually drinking the decoction of it helps red faces, tetters, and ringworms, because Mars causeth them. It helps the plague, sores, boils, and itch, the bitings of mad dogs [see also TREACLE] and venomous beasts, all which infirmities are under Mars. Thus you see what it does by sympathy.'

Thirst, Provoking
Nicholas Culpeper passed on the folk wisdom of the centuries: 'ONIONS. Mars owns them. They are flatulent and windy, and provoke appetite, increase thirst, ease the bowels, used with honey and rue.'

Tissicks
Not the cavalry of a newly independent republic, but coughs, either chin or chest, which see. The standard Real Medicine remedy for an annoying, tickly cough in a child was non-addictive and environmentally green:

> For an annoying tissick by a child, such as might render choleric a father who is about his sports, or a mother when she knitteth: Capture five Great and Hairy Spiders of the kind that frequenteth privies. Tie them loosely in a muslin bag or kerchief and suspend the live Creatures from the neck of the coughing child close beneath the chin. The Tissick shall soon cease.

Or, 'Take five common spiders and put them alive into an oven until they be charred. Sprinkle the ash of their bodies into a beaker of warm milk and give unto the childe to drink of, both morning and night.'

Parents who followed that advice found that it worked – the tickly cough cleared up in three or four days.

Tobacco
This noxious weed has had a mixed press over the centuries, being praised and cursed in equal measure, but the medical view has been more volatile than most. Back in the time when college medicine and hedgerow medicine roughly agreed about most plants, tobacco, like cannabis, was widely seen as a useful pharmaceutical tool. Dr

Thornton put the view of the fashionable physician in the eighteenth century:

> Tobacco is a well-known drug, of a narcotic quality, which it discovers in all persons, even in small quantity, when first applied to them. I have known a small quantity of it, snuffed up the nose, produce giddiness, stupor and vomiting; and when applied in different ways, in larger quantity, there are many instances of its more violent effects, even of its proving a mortal poison.

However, as we have already seen, he found that the nausea and giddiness known to many schoolboys could be bypassed, as it were, by anal insertions using a simple attachment or ordinary household bellows; this enabled him to fill a patient's bowels with soothing smoke with virtually no risk of lung cancer.

Unlit tobacco could be helpful, too, when doctors visited smelly, leaking children: 'Such as wait upon the sick in infantile diseases, run very great hazard. They ought to stuff their noses with tobacco or some other strong-smelling herb, as rue, tansy or the like.'

Toothache

The replacement of grinding drills by laser technology – especially if hard-tissue lasers become affordable – has taken some of the agony out of visits to the dentist. To avoid pain altogether, early readers of Mercellus Empiricus learned by heart some '*Incantamenta magica*', although the agony of suffering continued while they waited for an appointment, in this case with the moon: 'A charm against toothache was to repeat the words Argidam, margidam, sturgidam, seven times on a Tuesday or Thursday when the moon was waning.'

But for the scientist, objective observation was essential. For example, what made teeth ache? A fourteenth-century scientist recorded these observations:

> Toothache is caused by humours descending from the brain or rising from the stomach; the sure cure is bleeding in the first case, vomiting in the second. Tooth decay arises from the presence of worms in the mouth; this can be proved by sight, for when the teeth are washed with warm water, and water is poured into a vessel, the worms can be seen swimming about.

Fair enough, but the author of the thirteenth-century text book, *Practica*, knew that until dentists were invented, there was little to be done: 'Let the reader note that I do not deal with certain affections, such as ... chronic toothache ... because I think they are incurable.' Others of the same era had shrewder marketing skills: 'Frogs, pressed against decayed teeth, will make them [the teeth] fall out; particularly efficacious are the frogs of Provence.' Strange that Peter Mayle chose to keep this one tiny piece of Provencal arcana to himself, after revealing so much else that was pleasingly trivial.

Rural English wisdom was that chewing whole black pepper seeds 'helps the toothache', but more exotic was this sixteenth-century remedy for toothache: 'Write vpon a trencoir of wood H A Ab Hur Hurst Gebal then the parteis name, Efter Scraip away wt. a knyff all the voyells then all the rest.'

Dyer's *English Folk Lore* refers to a more recent oddity:

> This superstition was common some years ago in Derbyshire, where there was an odd way of extracting, as it was thought, the worm. A small quantity of a mixture consisting of dried and powdered herbs was placed in a teacup, and a live coke from the fire was dropped in. The patient then held his or her open mouth over the cup and inhaled the smoke as long as it could be borne. The cup was then taken away and a fresh cup or glass containing water was put before the patient. Into this cup the patient breathed hard for a few moments, and then, it was supposed, the grub or worm could be seen in the water.

So what did they see in the water? If there was nothing there, and the tooth still ached, the patient could sit beside an anthill and eat a crust of bread, then spit it out over the anthill, and as the ants ate the bread the tooth would cease to ache. Possibly. See also RABIES.

Travails, Easing

A useful obstetric cure-all was recommended by Nicholas Culpeper: '... the chymical oil drawn from the [*Juniperis Communis*] berries. They are good for the cough, shortness of breath, consumption, pains on the belly, ruptures, cramps, convulsions, and speedy delivery to pregnant women.' A dose of gin might have the same effect.

The traditional folk treatment for easing childbirth was Horehound (*Marrubium vulgare*), more widely known for centuries as a cough cure when mixed with sugar or as a fluid extract in doses of four to eight millilitres; but Nich. Culpeper swore by it as an obstetric aid: 'Horehound is a herb of Mercury. A decoction of the dried herb, and the seed, or the juice of the green herb taken with honey ... is given to women to bring down their courses, to expel the afterbirth, and to them that have sore and long travails.' Most women probably preferred this to surgical intervention in the blood-stained, septic hospitals of the day, but Culpeper, strongly influenced by astrological theories of planets and humours, added this caveat to the use of horehound: 'It should be used with caution, viz, that it ought only to be administered to gross phlegmatic persons, not to thin plethoric people.'

Travails – A Surgeon's View

The surgeon's approach to painful gynaecological conditions was put in 1839 by Dr Sharp[82]:

> Take leaves of hart's-tongue, Alchymilla, Pylosella, Plantago, Bugle, Tapsus Barbatus, of each 3 handfuls; rind of 4 Oranges. On all this pour 3 pints of whey. Distill in a common vessel.
>
> It is perhaps fitting to lessen the pain that she should sit in a perforated seat and draw into the affected parts the fumes evaporating from the hot decoction of this kind: Rx leaves of tapsus barbatus, 3 handfuls. Cook in spring water s.q.
>
> If pessaries can be used smear them with an ointment of populneum or linseed, or both mixed together and pounded till black in a lead mortar.
>
> But the best method of cure is to use milk or whey daily in large quantities, or (if obtainable) slightly acid waters, so long as they contain no pungency, like those drunk at Buxton in Derbyshire.
>
> Let her morning and evening drink ass's or cow's milk raw and mixed with the aforesaid distillation and sweetened with rose sugar or syrup of violets. At other times let her drink it cooked with bread or dehusked oats, adding a portion of spring water.

This was before orthodox and complementary practitioners parted company.

Treacle, Poor Man's

A treacle (Greek *theriake*, antidote to bite of wild beasts) was a prophylactic against bites and poisons, and the one that came readiest to hand in our ancient villages was garlic, according to Culpeper: 'Mars owns this herb. This was commonly accounted the poor man's treacle, it being a remedy for all diseases and hurts (except those which itself breeds). It helps the biting of mad dogs, and other venomous creatures.' This may well have worked, but garlic treacle as a spread would never have proved a threat to Tate and Lyle.

A prophylactic that was popular in the twelfth century had disappeared from the shelves by the thirteenth century, never to reappear; medical historians are baffled as to the reason for this, but biologists point to the gradual decline in the native wolf population: 'Write on the bark of a tree the formula given to you; tie the magical amulet upon your arm and recite the special prayers as you gather wolves' dung, mouse droppings, serpents' skins and cats' dung. Mix these with your own urine into your food and you will be proof against the onset of all diseases.'

Trephining

We turn to John Abernethy FRS and his observations in 1810:[83] his accounts cause one to believe that in those days anyone who could make a chair could make a surgeon:

> A man was knocked down by the iron hooks of a crane, which fell upon
> his head from a considerable height. He arrived senseless and deeply
> apoplectic. A fracture with depression was discovered, running
> obliquely across the anterior and inferior angle of the parietal bones,
> and over the temporal bone extending to the basis of the cranium,
> before the mastoid process.
>   Several perforations with the trephine were made along the course
> of the fracture and the depressed portion taken away. The brain, which
> had been indented by the pressure of congealed blood upon the dura
> mater, remained in the same state with little or no benefit from the
> operation, and he died within twelve hours after receiving the blow.

Apart from that, a thoroughly successful operation well worth
writing up. The most widespread use of trephining these days is to
relieve the pressure caused by subungual haematomata, or painful
bruises under a finger nail: one straightens out and heats a paper clip,
then drills it through the nail for immediate welcome relief from the
pressure.[84]

U

Ulcers

Also known as cankers, they are a sort of abscess brought on by such
ghastlinesses as general ill-health, gout, diabetes, varicose veins,
scurvy, syphilis and not washing. There were a lot of them about in
The Good Old Days. Mr Culpeper recommended an intrusive weed:
'The juice of alehoof [ground ivy], boiled in a little honey and
verdigris, stayeth the spreading of the cancers and ulcers.' Or there
was hedge mustard (*Sisymbrium Officinale*): 'It grows by the way and
hedge-sides, and sometimes in open fields. It is common in the Isle of
Ely. The juice made into a syrup with honey and sugar, is effectual
for coughs, wheezing and shortness of breath. The seed is good for
ulcers and cankers in the mouth, throat, or behind the ear.'
  The scarlet campion was an unlikely contender for defeating
ulcers, but it 'worked', given a favourable horoscope and a keen
sense of humours:

There are forty-five kinds of campion; those of them which are of a physical use having the like virtues with those above described, which I take to be the chiefest kinds ... They belong unto Saturn ... It is of very great use in old sores, ulcers, cankers, fistulas, and the like, to cleanse and heal them by consuming the moist humours falling into them, and correcting the putrefaction of humours offending them.

Ulcers, of the Bladder

Conventional medicine of the time had little to say about treating this problem, but Culpeper had some intriguing ideas based on the balance of humours that governed the body under the influence of various planets. A whole pseudo-science had built up over the centuries around this theory, such that there was even a chart of humorous temperatures, helping us to understand today why it is so important never to keep cucumbers in a refrigerator:

There is no dispute to be made but that they are under the dominion of the Moon, though they are so much cried out against for their coldness, and if they were but one degree colder they would be poison. The best of Galenists hold them to be cold and moist in the second degree, and then not so hot as lettuce or purslain [*Portulaca oleracea*].

There is not a better remedy growing for ulcers in the bladder than cucumbers are. The usual course is to use the seed in emulsions, as they make almond milk; but a far better way, in my opinion, is this: When the season of the year is, take the cucumbers and bruise them well and distil the water from them, and let such as are troubled with ulcers in the bladder drink no other drink.

Cucumbers also remedied hot rheums in the eyes, skin blemishes, pissing by drops, broken veins in the face, sun burn, freckles and morphew (which see). Such cosmetic treatments, highly processed and expensively packaged, are still widely sold.

Ulcers, Rotten & Filthy

The Cuckoo Pint was highly thought of for treating ulcers that had been allowed to deteriorate: 'The leaves either green or dry, or the juice of them, doth cleanse all manner of rotten and filthy ulcers, in what part of the body soever.' For really rotten and dreadfully filthy ulcers this might not be enough: 'The berries or roots beaten with hot ox-dung' could also be applied. There was a lot of dung in Real Medicine's heyday.

Ultra Sound Scans

A useful hint from a thirteenth-century gynaecologist on how to perform a body scan on a pregnant woman: 'Place a little vessel full of water on her breast; if it moves, she is alive, but if not, she is dead.'

Nowadays, the diagnostics are usually connected to high-tech computer software rather than to the patient's own natural software.

V

Variolation

When Lady Montague was on holiday in Turkey in 1718 she observed an intriguing local custom, and described it in a letter to her friends at home, thereby introducing in one go two admirable ideas, inoculation against smallpox, and interesting holiday postcards. This inoculation, however, did not involve surgical spirit or sterile syringes:

> The small-pox, so fatal and general amongst us, is here entirely harmless, by the invention of *ingrafting*, which is the term they give it. There is a set of old women who make it their business to perform the operation every autumn, in the month of September, when the great heat is abated. People send to one another to see if any of their family has a mind to have the small-pox; they make parties for this purpose, and when they are met (commonly fifteen or sixteen together), the old woman comes with a nut-shell full of the matter of the best sort of small-pox, and asks what vein you please to have opened.
>
> She immediately rips open the one that you offer to her with a large needle (which gives you no more pain than a common scratch), and puts into the vein as much matter as can lie upon the head of her needle, and after that binds up the little wound with a hollow bit of shell, and in this manner opens four or five veins.
>
> Every year thousands undergo this operation; and the French ambassador says pleasantly, that they take the small-pox here by way of diversion, as they take the waters in other countries. There is no example of any that has died in it; and you may believe that I am well satisfied of the safety of this experiment, since I intend to try it on my own little son.'

Her son survived the experiment, and when she returned to England later in 1718, she set vigorously about introducing the ancient practice properly called variolation [*variola*, a blotch]. She took pus from a vesicle on a local suffering from a mild form of smallpox and scraped it into the skin of her young son, thereby inoculating him. She did the same for her infant daughter during an outbreak in London, and the child survived. Soon the royal family wondered whether their princes should be protected, but it was first tried out on 'several criminals and orphan children', and when even these expendables survived, the princes were also inoculated, or variolated.

Soon there were Real Medicine variolaters throughout the country, mainly elderly women, as in Turkey. This caused problems for the early chambers of commerce. A Nimby butcher or draper would not like to have several dozen poxy peasants coming to his next-door neighbour's house for treatment each day, discouraging trade, so they got organized:

Colchester, May 12, 1762.

The Practice of bringing people out of the country into this town to be inoculated for the Small-pox being very prejudicial to the town in many respects, but especially to the Trade thereof, and as by this practice the distemper may be continued much longer in the town than it otherwise would, in all probability, it is thought proper by some of the principal inhabitants and traders in the town, that this public notice should be given that they are determined to prosecute any person or persons whomsoever, that shall hereafter bring into this town, or who shall receive into their houses in the town as lodgers, any person or persons for that purpose, with the utmost severity that the law will permit ... But that they might not be thought discouragers of the practice so salutary and beneficial to mankind, as inoculation is found to be, which encourages great numbers to go into the practice, the persons who have caused this public notice to be given have no objection to surgeons carrying on the practice in houses properly situated for the purpose.[85]

It was unlikely that many surgeons would oblige, for the British medical establishment opposed inoculation as yet another old wives' tale. The public was unimpressed; advertisements for servants and apprenticeships around the years 1760–80 listed a pox-marked face as the most desirable of assets, though being dull, dowdy and overweight would also help:

WANTED, in a large family, a STOUT WOMAN, about 30, single, or a widow without children, who has had the Small-pox, to take care of a lusty child, under a year old. Her character must be unexceptionable, and by no means a fashionable dresser, and lived in families of credit. Any person answering this description may enquire of MRS MERCER, at the Star and Garter, Andover, and be further informed.

Wanted an Apprentice to an eminent Surgeon in full practice in the county of Suffolk. If he has not had the Small-Pox, it is expected he will be inoculated for it, before he enters on business. – Enquire of JOHN FOX, at Dedham, Essex.

In the newly independent United States it was a great success, with thousands successfully variolated in their new hospitals, like the Pennsylvania Hospital of Philadelphia (1751) and the New York Hospital (1791).

The official death rate from smallpox in London in Lady Montagu's time was four thousand per million. Edward Jenner, a pupil of the Dr Hunter after whom syphilis symptoms were named, successfully experimented on young James Phipps in 1796 after a twenty-year evaluation of the process, then wrote '*An Inquiry into the Causes and Effects of the Variolae Vaccinae*': this helped to make vaccination medically respectable at last. In 1803 the Royal Jannerian Society was formed with Royal patronage to move the process along. Then, in 1804, an Act of Parliament outlawed it. In 1805 the Lord Chancellor carried a motion in the House of Commons that the Royal College of Physicians be required to inquire and report on the progress of vaccination. In 1806 the Jannerians changed their name to the National Vaccination Institute, and the RCP reported that 'within eight years of the discovery of vaccination some hundreds of thousands had been vaccinated in the British Islands, and upwards of 800,000 in our East Indian possessions, and that the practice had been generally adopted in Europe'. Smallpox, they reported, destroyed one-sixth of those it attacked, and nearly one-tenth of the entire mortality of London was caused by it.

Acting urgently in the light of this damning report, Parliament rushed through the Vaccination Act a mere thirty-four years later. This Act effectively took the business away from old ladies and gave it to the doctors. In 1853 it was made compulsory for those travelling abroad. By the 1970s vaccination [Latin, *vacca*, a cow] had apparently eliminated smallpox worldwide. In the 1980s, mass vaccination with infected needles was being speculatively linked to the spread of AIDS, the new scourge that seems set to take the place of smallpox.

While the official view see-sawed, the country's mothers made their own decisions, according to Dr Buchan's prescient remarks in 1794:

Few mothers, some years ago, would submit to have their children inoculated even by the hand of a Physician; yet nothing is more certain than that of late many of them have performed this operation with their own hand; and as their success has been equal to that of the most dignified inoculators, there is little reason to doubt that the practice will become general. Whenever this shall be the case, more lives will be saved by inoculation alone, than are at present by all the endeavours of the Faculty.

Until well into this century inoculation was performed by scarifying the upper arm with a cut-throat razor; in Buchan's day pus from a cow-pox vesicle would be collected and scraped into the skin. He added a comment that helps lay people understand the difficult relationship between a professional organization that dislikes self-promotion and a widely published medical author: 'Very few of the valuable discoveries in Medicine have been made by physicians. They have generally either been the effect of chance or of necessity, and have generally been opposed by the Faculty, till everyone else was convinced of their importance.'

The Faculty (BMA) certainly did not like doctors who went into print, so Dr Buchan, who went into print like billy-o, did not like the Faculty; this coloured his view of his senior colleagues to some extent. There was some substance, however, in his charge that the profession was over-cautious in its attitude to vaccination.

Venery, or Venereal Diseases

Let's start with blame. The classical British name for syphilis was Morbus Gallicus – the French Disease, or the French pox. But it had not always been so. In Andrew Boord's *Breviary of Helthe* of 1547 there is first of all the blame – Who gave us Spanish Flu? Dutch Elm Disease? German Measles? Danish Blue? Then he lists all the forms of syphilis that he knew, relentlessly adding detail to detail until everyone knew more than they wanted to know about pockes and was well and truly bored: on the other hand, it makes an appealing monologue for recitation at parties and functions:

> In englyshe Morbus Gallicus is named the franch pockes, whan that I was yonge they were named the spanyshe pockes the which be of many kind of pockes, some be moyst, some be waterashe, some be drye, and some be skorvie, some be lyke scabbes, some be lyke ring wormes, some be fistuled, some be festered, some be cankarus, some be like wennes, some be lyke byles, some be lyke knobbes or burres, and some be ulcerous havyinge a lytle dry skabbe in the midst of the ulcerous skabbe, some hath ache in the jointes and no sign of the pockes, and yet it may be the pockes …
>
> The cause of these impediments or infyrmytes doth come many ways, it maye come by lyenge in the shetes or bedde where a pocky person hath the night before been lyenin, it may come with lyenge with a pocky person, it maybe come by syttenge oft with a pocky person, it may come by syttenge on a draught or sege [privy], it maye come by drynkynge oft with a pocky person, but specially is it taken when one

pocky person doth synn in lechery the one with another. All the kinds of pockes be infectiouse.

An amazingly high percentage of syphilis cases came from 'syttenge on a sege', one suspects, and hardly any from 'lechery the one with another'. Dr Buchan in 1776 was very terse about lechery, blaming it entirely on men: 'Some men make love for amusement, others from mere vanity, or on purpose to show their consequence with the fair. This is perhaps the greatest piece of cruelty which one can be guilty of.' How widespread was venereal disease? How many pocky people were there? A report from St Bartholomew's Hospital in 1554 said of syphilitics: 'Among every twentye diseased persons that are taken in, fiftene of them have the pocks. The filthye type of many lewd and idell persons, both men and women about the citye of London, and the great number of lewd alehouses, which are the very nests and harbourers of such filthy creatures.' Treatment was trickier to define. In 1587 it was believed that syphilis could be cured by immersion in the Bath waters (q.v.).

The moment that Dr Buchan's patients dreaded was when he uttered his dread diagnosis and wrote out his dread prescription:

For gonorrhoea (that which recurs frequently is called The Gleets; if buboes occur in the groin, it is the Confirmed Lues,) apply the blue ointment, that which is made by rubbing together equal quantities of hogs' lard and quicksilver; about a drachm may be used at time, and the most proper place is the inner side of the thigh.

The treatment? Clearly, human wickedness had to be punished while the symptoms were being allayed: 'With The Gleets the treatment should be often repeated, and accompanied by the last remedy that we shall mention, the cold bath. Alternatively, take half a drachm of mercurial pill night and morning, or mercury may be taken in a liquid form, as it is suspended in a watery mixture.'

The recipe for the mercureal bolus was simple enough to be made up in the householder's own scullery:

Make a diaphonetic mercureal bolus thus: take of calomel [not caramel, but the subchloride of mercury; not as deadly a poison as perchloride of mercury], six grains; conserve of roses, half a drachm; make a bolus thereof, and take over night with a glass of mercury [the vagueness as to quantities with this toxic heavy metal might disturb some present-day physicians] in watery mixture.

For abscess, gangrene, cancer, ulcer and chances [shallow ulcers], mercury is the only confirmed cure of these diseases.

Another rigorous treatment for venereal diseases was Dr Buchan's mercurial plaster: 'Take of common plaster one pound; of gum ammoniac, strained, a half pound. Melt them together, and, when cooling, add eight ounces of quicksilver, previously extinguished by triture with three ounces of hogs' lard.'

There seems little doubt that these Real Medicine treatments for gonorrhoea and syphilis shortened the sufferer's pains, like this mainstream advice of 1778:

> Take of sarsaparilla three ounces; of liquorice and mezerion root, half an ounce; of crude antimony [a poison that can paralyse the heart and nervous system; in smaller quantities it makes you cough, empty your bowels and sweat, often in that order], powdered, one and a half grains. Infuse these ingredients in eight pints of water for twenty four hours, then boil till one half of the boiling water is consumed; afterwards, strain the decoction. It strengthens and restores flesh and vigour to parts emaciated by the venereal disease. Take with a few glasses of mercury.

The mercury would be a problem to our modern mind; it would probably be unlawful to bury the patient within ten miles of any water source.

Dr Buchan also treated gonorrhoea: 'Take of senna, coriander, tamarinds, French prunes mixed with syrup of sugar, rhubarb powder and nitre in a decoction. Take a drachm, about the bulk of a nutmeg, during the inflammation and tension of the urinary passages, which accompany a virulent gonorrhoea.' As a palliative, herbalists suggested a discreet dab of ground ivy: 'Add alehoof to white wine, and some honey and a little burnt alum, it is excellent, guaranteed to wash the sores and ulcers in the privy parts of man or woman.'

VD & the Prime Minister's Scalp

When Lord Melton, the Prime Minister in June 1742, went down with gonorrhoea, they sent for Dr Pye and Dr Logan.[86] Blotches would appear on the PM's scalp and then burst – possibly during Prime Minister's Questions. The doctors did the obvious thing, prescribing chopped-up gall stones from a goat – 'Beazor's mineral' – followed by Viper Broth and Bristol Water, none of which 'worked'. They then tried: 'an electuary consisting of three ounces of emollient, three drams of powdered julep, a half of purified nitre, bound together with lemon juice, taken twice a day'. This worked to the doctors' complete satisfaction, though with an 'however' from the PM: 'The dark greenish poison was slowly oozing from his penis, which was all contracted, and the sharp and constant pain extended from the perineum up to the urinary bladder, producing small swellings now in this place and now in that.' They suggested that he 'bathe the part in tepid water and milk, applying poultices [not during Prime Minister's Questions], and a few grains of laudanum at night'. He died, of course, leaving this ability to ooze dark green poison from his penis as his only claim to fame.

Culpeper's *Complete Herbal* suggested boiling the fleshy tops of hops when they were ripe in August and drinking the juice, for 'it cures the venereal disease'. Then, as now, the sufferer had the choice, but a little-known Culpepery fact is that: 'Sea holly is venereal, under the celestial Balance. It cures French pox and pissing by drops.'

Another of his favoured plants was the Holy Thistle, whose use was recommended with irresistible clinical logic: 'By antipathy to other planets it cureth the French Pox. By antipathy to Venus, who governs it, it strengthens the memory, and cures deafness by antipathy to Saturn, who hath his fall in Aries, which rules the head.'

Venice Treacle

Sir Ralph and Lady Verney were visiting Venice in 1651 when they discovered an interesting medicine, which they sent home to their friend Mrs Isham, for her family medicine chest with the warning that some of its contents might upset her tender tummy, for 'honey disagrees with some particular constitutions'; this was possibly a joke, in very nasty taste:

> Hee that is most famous for treacle is Sig Antonio Sgobis, and keeps shoppe at the Strazzo, or Ostridge, on the right hand going towards St Mark's. His price is 19 livres (Venize money) apound, and hee gives leaden Potts with the Ostridge signe uppon them, and papers both Italian and Lattin to show its virtue.
>
> It was traditionally composed by Nero's physician, and was made of vipers, white wine, and opium, spices from both the Indies, liquorice, red roses, tops of germander, juice of rough aloes, seeds of treacle mustard [now produced in the famed treacle mines of West Cornwall], tops of St John's wort, and some twenty other herbs, to be mixed with honey triple the weight of the dry species into an electuary.
>
> Vipers are essential, and to get the full value of them, a dozen vipers should be put alive into the white wine. Venice treacle may be as well made in England, though their country is hotter, and so may the more rarify the viperime juices, yet the bites of our vipers at the proper time of the year, which is the hottest, are as efficacious and deadly as them.

There were warnings against overdosing on this opiate nastiness, yet it was still being described as late as 1739 in Dr Quincey's *English Dispensatory*. What tough people our forebears were.

Wambling Trots, the, See **quacks,** *diseases not yet known to mankind ...*

Waterloo Teeth

The problem with making false teeth was that human saliva dissolves almost anything given time – look at beefburgers. Keeping the top set in place was another problem. French women of the sixteenth and early seventeenth centuries even had steel hooks piercing their gums in order to hold their false teeth in place. Then, in the early seventeenth century, a Parisian dentist called Fauchard 'fastened the upper and lower sets with steel springs'. This kept the upper teeth secure but meant that the ladies in question had to keep their mouths clamped shut at other times. They did not like this.

Human teeth pulled from a 'donor' and poked into a recent cavity in the recipient's mouth sometimes worked, but the trick was to get enough 'donors'.

Then along came Napoleon, starting wars he couldn't finish, especially the Battle of Waterloo. The result? Lots of dead bodies with lots of lovely redundant teeth – hence the old proverb, 'Dead men chew no rope'. Many an ageing Regency dandy was happy to have his stained or rotted teeth removed and a few 'Waterloos' popped in as replacements. The American Civil War helped dentists, too: teeth taken from corpses, whether or not they carried a valid donor card, were removed and shipped to Britain by the barrelful to meet a constant demand.[87]

Weak, Watery, Bleared Eyes

The Anglo-Saxon Leech Book took a firm view: 'Take a live crab, put his eyes out, and put him alive again into the water, and put the eyes upon the neck of the man who hath need. He will soon be well.' The RSPCA was not founded until 1824.

According to Foulsham & Co's early reprint of Culpeper's

Complete Herbal: 'The juice of the herb [Honey Wort, *Cerinthe Major*] with a little saffron dissolved in it, is an excellent remedy for weak, watery, bleared eyes, when used instead of Bugloss and Borage.' An alternative was Horehound (*Marubium Vulgare*): 'The juice, with wine and honey, helps clear the eyesight.'

For those lacking faith in medicine, a glazier trading in Italy between 1280 and 1285 made some 'glass lentils', simple lenses (lens = *lente*, Italian for lentil) that could be held close to the eye for better vision. They did not catch on.

Whooping Cough

Known two or three hundred years ago as a chin cough, and now professionalized as pertussis, it is a one-off illness of childhood. Traditional treatment was no different from that for a chest cough, on a suck-it-and-see basis, but the *Pall Mall Gazette* of 12 October 1866 carried a horrid story of one cure that went wrong:

> At an inquest held on the fifth of October, at Bradfield (Bucks) on the body of a child of five years, which had died of hydrophobia, evidence was given of a practice almost incredible in civilised England. Sarah Mackness stated that at the request of the mother of the deceased, she had fished out of the river the body of the dog by which the child had been bitten, and had extracted its liver, a slice of which she had frizzled before the fire, and had then given it to the child to be eaten with some bread. The dog had been drowned nine days before. The child ate the liver greedily, drank some tea afterwards, but died in spite of this strange specific.

The most surprising detail of that story was perhaps the use of the expression 'in spite of'. Not recommended.

In their book *Homeopathy for Doctor and Patient*,[88] two French homeopathists explained their approach:

> As everyone knows, whooping-cough is caused by Bordet Gengou's bacillus [*Bordetella pertussis*], which is characterised by paroxysms of the distinctive coughing ... Unable to destroy the microbe responsible, we were reduced to using medicines chosen completely at random in an attempt to alleviate the symptoms. The parents of the sufferers often gave old wives' remedies, such as, for example, the slime of a snail, chosen on the principle of analogy – this substance resembles the strands of phlegm coughed up by a child, the doctrine of signatures, often confused with homeopathy.

After various experiments, they settled on Drosera, Belladonna and Coccus cacti as the homeopathic response to whooping cough. Dr Buchan had a specific prescription for a chin cough – his popular

Decoction of Alcthen; this is how he dispensed it in 1776: 'Take of the roots of the marsh mallow moderately dried, three ounces; raisins of the sun, one ounce; water, three pints. Boil the ingredients in water till one third of it is consumed; then strain the decoction and let it stand for some time to settle. The decoction is used for an ordinary drink when coughing.'

Witchcraft

Now largely the province of covens of social workers, witchcraft was once considered a health threat to be taken seriously. Mr Culpeper's herbal remedy used the woody nightshade, or bitter sweet (*Solanum dulcamara*): 'It is under the planet Mercury and a notable herb of his also, if it be rightly gathered under his influence. Good also to remove witchcraft in men and beasts, as also all sudden diseases whatsoever.'

Womb, Trouble with the

A worried general practitioner wrote in the 1670s to Dr Thomas Willis[89] for advice on treating a patient with a severe uterine disorder called 'phlogosis [Greek *phlogizein*, to burn], with intense torture'; from his detailed description it might even have been cancer. Dr Willis agonized over her fate before offering his professional advice:

> The Curative intentions are very narrowly confined and comprise practically only these two aims, namely to sweeten the blood and meanwhile to draw off its wastes and dregs, from the affected parts. Phlebotomy from the veins of the arms is to be used, and serves both intentions. And in a similar case I have known the following remedy to bring great help, namely that every month or six weeks up to 5 or 6ozs of blood should be let.
> If a draught of whey, with infused flowers of pale Roses and correctives, suit her, exhibit it every 7th or 10th day; or if through queasiness of the stomach Medicines are required in very small quantity I would prescribe pills of this sort, which contain nothing deleterious:
> Best Senna 1 oz, Rhubarb 6 drachms, lemon sandal 1 drachm, salt of Absynth ½ drachm, yellow Oranges 1 drachm; cut and pound. Infuse lukewarm in water of Fumaria ¾ pint for 12 hours. Strain. Evaporate to an extract in a very gently heated Bath, adding towards the end best Senna powdered 2 drachms, Rhubarb powder 1½ drachms, lemon sandal 1 drachm. Make a mass and form into pills. Dose 2 scruples to ½ drachm.
> Prepare this sort of distilled water, of which she is to take 3 to 4 ozs, twice or thrice a day, sweetened with Syrup, stuck on a pin and imbued with powder of white sugar.

One hopes it helped the poor woman.

Women Newly Brought to Bed

All you need to know is that they have to be cleansed. Here is how to do it herbally; doctors probably used mercury:

> Take a pound of wood and leaves [of woody nightshade] together, bruise the wood, then put in a pot, and put into it three pints of white wine; put on the pot lid and shut it close; and let it infuse hot over a gentle fire twelve hours, and then strain it out ... to cleanse women newly brought to bed.[90]

But *Medical History* (Vol 32 no 3 July 1988) also caught the cold disregard that many male doctors had for their female patients, some of whom even feared having lancets cutting into their breasts. Women! Huh!

> Women in childbed often commit the cure of their inflamed breasts to their nurses, or to some doting old woman; and as they fear nothing more than a suppuration, and an opening of the suppurating parts by the surgeon's lancet, they therefore use all their endeavours to prevent it ... they, by a dangerous error, expose the inflamed breast to the heat of a burning coal, or else continually foment it with very dry and hot linen cloths, or else they apply spirit of wine almost scalding, by which means, instead of suppuration following, the more fluid parts are exhaled, and the rest of the matter is inspissated into an irresolvable schirrus; and then the unhappy woman who was so much afraid of a slight puncture from a sharp lancet, is frequently obliged afterwards to undergo the very severe and dangerous operation of amputating.

Inspissated means 'a failure to disperse an internal collection of material, expulsion of morbid matter from the body'. The poor women who tried natural ways to avoid agonizing surgery were, it seems, told it was all their own silly fault when they finally faced a fearsome mastectomy. However, if the problem was in becoming pregnant, old wives were as full of advice as the hedges were of nostrums: 'Try eating the leaves of wild pansies [*viola tricolor*, or heartsease]. Ivy leaves are rarely known to fail. The greater periwinkle [*Vinca minor* or *Vinca major*, but not *Littorina littorea*, an edible gastropod].

Worms

If worms caused your loss of appetite, you could try out this Anthelminthic [worm-killing] Wine on someone: 'Take of rhubarb, half an ounce; worm seed, an ounce. Bruise them, and infuse without heat in two pints of red port wine for a few days. Strain off the wine and take a glass two or three times a day. Or reduce to a powder, which also kills the worms.'[91]

Woundwort, or All-Heal

Mr Culpeper was not too fond of animal-based cures, preferring broad-spectrum nostrums based on English-grown plants, one of his favourite of which was All-heal or Woundwort [*Valeriana officinalis*]. Its rhizomes and roots, as you probably know, produce valerianic acid [$C_5H_{10}O_2$] in several isomers, as well as a volatile oil that is believed to act as a sedative on the nervous system, but Culpeper made such sweeping claims for it that a herbalist could probably have made a living trading in this one plant alone:

> It is under the dominion of Mars, hot, biting and cholerick; and remedies what evils Mars afflicts the body of man with, by sympathy, as the loadstone, iron.
>   It kills the worms, helps the gout, cramp and convulsions, provokes urine, and helps all joint-aches. It helps all cold griefs of the head, the vertigo, falling sickness, and the lethargy.

And almost everything else, including 'every ague soever'.

Yellow Emperor's Classic of Internal Medicine

A person who is unwell but lacks confidence in orthodox medicine, herbalism or lumbar-crunching could look back 2,300 years to this treatise on traditional Taoist thinking, as did Edward de Bono when editing his oeuvre, *Eureka! How & when the Greatest Inventions were made*. The body is divided along twelve vertical meridians along which, they then thought, were 365 points at which needling would produce a physiological effect; current acupuncturists have located 800 such points that tap into the aspects of the universe that are stored in three regions of the abdomen. They see their intervention as helping to keep these universal forces in perfect balance.

    The main claimed effect of acupuncture was to drive out harmful secretions: in this at least it was similar to most therapies over the ages. The fact that needling permits a patient to undergo surgery while fully awake still puzzles western practitioners, because, while acupuncture undoubtedly 'works', it ought not to.

Yellow Jaundice & Black Jaundice

From the French *jaunisse, jaunir* – to become yellow. Woody nightshade (*Amara dulcis* – now *solanum dulcamara*) was widely used, according to Culpeper:

> Take a pound of wood and leaves together, bruise the wood, then put in a pot, and put into it three pints of white wine; put on the pot lid and shut it close; and let it infuse hot over a gentle fire twelve hours, and then strain it out, so you have a most excellent drink to open obstructions of the liver and spleen, to help difficulty of breath, bruises and falls, and congealed blood in any part of the body; it helps a yellow jaundice, the dropsy, and the black jaundice.

There was also Horehound (*Marubium Vulgare*), especially useful for patients with large nostrils and an earache: 'The juice, with wine and honey, snuffed up the nostrils, it purges away the yellow jaundice; and, with oil of roses, dropped into the ears, eases the pain of them.' See also **King's Evil.**

Z

Zodiac & Health

We had one of four humours dominant, according to the zodiac school of etiology: we were either sanguine, choleric, phlegmatic or melancholic, and there was nothing we could do about it. The astrologer, with his arcane mysteries from ancient Babylon, taught that our humours were fixed by the relationship between his punters and the stars; the zodiac controlled the outward body, while the planets the inner organs and fluids. Roughly equivalent to Freudian psychology.

References

1. *Medical History*, vol 18, 1974. The Wellcome Institute for the History of Medicine
2. *The English Physician Enlarged* or 'The Herbal, with Three Hundred & Sixty-Nine Medicines made of English Herbs that were not in any Impression until This, Being an Astrologo-Physical Discourse of the Vulgar Herbs of this Nation, containing a complete Method of Physic, whereby a Man may preserve his Body in Health, or cure Himself, being Sick, for Three-Pence Charge, with such Things only as grow in England, they being most fit for English Bodies,' by Nich. Culpeper, Gent, Student in Physic & Astrology, 1653. Reprinted in Berwick 1801 and thereafter
3. Brian Inglis and Ruth West, *The Alternative Health Guide*, (Michael Joseph, London 1983)
4. *Mémoires de la Société Royale de Médecine*, Paris 1806, Vol. 8, page 310: 'Reflétions sur le Traitement de la manie Atrabilaire comparé a celui de Plusieurs autres Maladies chroniques, et sur l'Avantage de la Méthode evacuante,' par M. Hallé
5. Ibid., page 70
6. Roderick E. McGrew, *Encyclopedia of Medical History*
7. *Mémoires de la Société Royale de Médecine*, Paris 1806
8. William Buchan MD, *Domestic Medicine Modernised*, 1808
9. Joseph Hume Spry, *A Practical Treatise on the Bath Waters, Tending to illustrate their beneficial Effects in Chronic Diseases, particularly in Gout, Rheumatism, Paralysis, Lead Colic, Indigestion, Biliary Affections, and Uterine & Cutaneous Diseases; confirmed by Cases*, Longmans, 13s
10. Ibid.
11. Robert John Thornton MD, Uni Camb, RLC Phys, *A Family Herbal, or familiar account of The Medical Properties of British & Foreign Plants, also Their Uses in Dying, and the Various Arts, arranged According to the Linnaean System*, London 1814
12. *Culpeper's Complete Herbal: Consisting of a Comprehensive Description of nearly all Herbs with their Medicinal Properties & Directions for compounding the Medicines extracted from them*, London, Foulsham & Co
13. John Abernethy FRS, *Surgical Observations on the Constitutional Origin & Treatment of Local Diseases, & on Aneurisms*, London, 1825
14. Roderick E. McGrew, *Encyclopedia of Medical History*
15. John Wesley, *The Desideratum: or, electricity made Plain and Useful. By a Lover of Mankind, and of Common Sense*, London 1760
16. *Medical History*

17. W.A.R. Thomson (ed.), *Black's Medical Dictionary*, 29th edition, London 1971
18. Thornton's *Herbal*, 1810
19. Acts 15:1–21; and Acts 21:25
20. 'Texts and Documents – some letters of Dr Thomas Willis (1621–1675)' by Kenneth Dewhurst
21. 'Blood transfusions were associated with infectious complications when given pre-, intra-, or post-operatively … The risk of postoperative infection increased progressively with the number of units of blood given.' *The British Journal of Surgery*, August 1988
22. *The New Encyclopedia Britannica*, Vol. 2, Macropaedia, 15th edition, 1985
23. Dr Michael Canquelin, *How Cosmic and Atmospheric Energies Influence Your Health*, Librairie Hachette, Paris 1967; translated by Stein & Day Inc, New York, 1971
24. Ibid., page 37
25. Joe Graedon and Teresa Graedon, *The People's Pharmacy*, St Martin's Press, New York, 1985
26. *Medical History*, 'The 1832 Cholera Epidemic in York, Margaret C. Barnet
27. Ibid.
28. Ibid.
29. John B. Keane, *Love Bites & Other Stories*, The Mercier Press, Cork, 1991
30. *Medical History*, Vol. 29, No. 4, October 1985: 'Medicine and pharmacy in British political prints', by William H. Helfand, New Jersey
31. William Birken PhD, 'The Social Problem of the English Physician in the early 17th century'
32. John Nicholls, *Literary Anecdotes of the Eighteenth Century*, Vol. 2
33. *Medical History*, Vol. 31, No. 2, April 1987: 'Health and Virtue; or, How to keep out of harm's way', by Rosalie Stott
34. *The People's Pharmacy*
35. Dr John Brisbane MD, *Selected Cases in the Treatment of Medicine*, London
36. W. van Barneveld, 'Geneeskundige electricteit' 3 vols, Amsterdam 1785–1789, i, 56f
37. W.D. Hackman, 'The Researches of Dr Martinus Van Marum (1750–1837) on the influence of electricity on animals and plants,' ibid.
38. J. Priestley, 'Experiments & Observations on Different Kinds of Air', 3 volumes, London, 1771–7; Vol. I, Section VIII
39. *Medical History*, Volume XVI, 1972. Ed. F.N.L. Poynter PhD, D. Litt, FRSL, FLA
40. Ibid., page 13
41. J. Priestley, *The History & Present State of Electricity*, London, 1767, Section XIV
42. Published by W. Foulsham & Co, Slough
43. Buchan, 1808
44. Dr John Abernethy FRS, 'Surgical Observations on the Constitutional Origin & Treatment of Local Diseases & on Aneurisms,' London 1825

45. Dr Trevor Smith MA MB B Chir DPM MFHom, *The Side-Effects Book ... what your doctor didn't have time to tell you*, Worthing 1989
46. *Medical History*, Vol. 30, No. 2, April 1986
47. Thornton's *Herbal*, 1810
48. Ibid., Introduction, page vii
49. Garfield Tourney, 'The Physician and Witchcraft in Restoration England'
50. William Buchan MD, *Domestic Medicine, or, a Treatise on the Prevention & Cure of Diseases by Regimen & Simple Medicines*, 5th Edition, 1776
51. William A.R. Thomson MD, *Black's Medical Dictionary*, 1951 edition
52. Richard Mabey (ed.), *The Complete New Herbal – a practical guide to herbal living*, Elm Tree Books, London, 1988
53. *Black's Medical Dictionary*, 1971 edition
54. Wm Andrews FRHS, *The Doctor in History, Literature & Folk Lore*, Hull 1896
55. *Medical History*, Vol. XVI, 1972
56. *Medical History*, Vol. 30, No. 2, April 1986, 'George Baker' by Gustav Ungerer
57. *The Complete New Herbal*
58. Thornton's *Family Herbal*, 1814
59. Ibid., page 527
60. *Medical History*, Vol. 30, No. 3, July 1986
61. William Buchan MD, *Domestic Medicine*, 1st edition
62. Ibid.
63. *Encyclopedia of Medical History*
64. William Buchan MD
65. John Abernethy FRS, 'Surgical Observations on Injuries to the Head & on Miscellaneous Subjects', London 1810
66. 'Texts and Documents – some letters of Dr Thomas Willis (1621–1675)'
67. Roderick E. McGrew, *Encyclopedia of Medical History*
68. *A Pictorial History of Medicine*
69. *Medical History*, 'The 1832 Cholera Epidemic in York', Margaret C. Barnet, 1972
70. Wm Andrews, *The Doctor*, 1896
71. Ibid.
72. 'Rabies in the Talmud' by Fred Rosner, Director of Hematology, Queens Hospital Center, NY, commenting on Yoma 84a and the Babylonian Talmud (*Shabbath* 121b)
73. William Buchan MD, *Domestic Medicine Modernised*, 1808
74. 'An Essay on the Medical Efficacy and employment of the Bath Waters', 1825
75. 'An Account of Two Successful Operations for Restoring a Lost Nose, from the Integuments of the Forehead, in the Cases of Two Officers of His Majesty's Army, including Descriptions of the Indian and Italian Methods,' by J.C. Carpue FRS, Longmans, London, 1802
76. Felix Marti-Ibanez MD (ed.), *A Pictorial History of Medicine*, Spring Books, London 1965
77. Dr John Brisbane, *Selected Cases in the Practice of Medicine*
78. Robert John Thornton, *A Family Herbal*, London, 1814
79. *Domestic Medicine Modernized*, 1808

80. John Abernethy FRS, *Surgical Observations*, London, 1825
81. *Medical History*, Vol. 30, No. 3, July 1986
82. 'A Practical Treatise on Wounds and other Chirurgical Subjects to which is affixed a short Historical Account of the Rise and Progress of Surgery and Anatomy addressed to young Surgeons; Vol. 2', London 1839
83. John Abernethy, 1810
84. According to Mr C.C. Scott, Consultant in Accident and Emergency Medicine, Southport and Formby District General Hospital, in a letter to *The Independent* on 28 February 1991
85. William Andrews FRHS, *The Doctor*, Hull, 1896
86. *Medical History*, Vol. 34, No. 2, April 1990: 'In Spite of Help: the Puzzle of an Eighteenth-Century Prime Minister's Illness,' by Marjorie Bloz
87. Edward de Bono (ed.), *Eureka! How and When the Greatest Inventions were Made*, Thames & Hudson, 1974
88. Michel Philippe and Aubin Picard, *Homeopathy for Doctor and Patient*, published in translation by Ashgrove Press, Bath, 1983
89. 'Texts and Documents – Some Letters of Dr Thomas Willis (1621–1675)' by Kenneth Dewhurst
90. Culpeper
91. Buchan, 1776